Lecture Notes of the Institute for Computer Sciences, Social Informatics and Telecommunications Engineering   118

Constantinos T. Angelis
Dimitrios Fotiadis
Alexandros T. Tzallas (Eds.)

Ambient Media and Systems

Third International ICST Conference
AMBI-SYS 2013
Athens, Greece, March 15, 2013
Revised Selected Papers

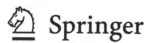 Springer

Volume Editors

Constantinos T. Angelis
Technological Educational Institute of Epirus
Kostakioi, Arta, Greece
E-mail: kangelis@teiep.gr

Dimitrios Fotiadis
University of Ioannina, Ioannina, Greece
E-mail: fotiadis@cc.uoi.gr

Alexandros T. Tzallas
University of Ioannina, Ioannina, Greece
E-mail: atzallas@cc.uoi.gr

ISSN 1867-8211   e-ISSN 1867-822X
ISBN 978-3-319-04101-8   e-ISBN 978-3-319-04102-5
DOI 10.1007/978-3-319-04102-5
Springer Cham Heidelberg New York Dordrecht London

Library of Congress Control Number: 2013955917

CR Subject Classification (1998): C.3, C.2, K.4, C.5, J.3, H.4, H.5

Typesetting: Camera-ready by author, data conversion by Scientific Publishing Services, Chennai, India

Printed on acid-free paper

Springer is part of Springer Science+Business Media (www.springer.com)

Preface

The tremendous advantages in mobile communications and mobile computing combined with the rapid evolution in smart appliances and devices, sensor-actuator technology, virtual environments, and interactive computing have generated new challenges and problems requiring interactions between different computer and communication technologies and applications in order to offer an unprecedented level of convenience and flexibility for living and working. Such technologies need to be closely integrated with human interactions and activity, allowing greater support for smart solutions that improve quality of life, productivity, understanding, and intelligence within their environment. They represent the vision of an all-encompassing multimedia networking environment with human interaction at its core.

AMBI-SYS 2013 addressed these areas and focused on emerging technologies, services, and solutions for new, human-centric intelligent ambient environments.

November 2013   Constantinos T. Angelis

Organization

General Chair

Constantinos T. Angelis   Technological Educational Institute of Epirus, Greece

Technical Program Committee Chair

Kanav Kahol   Arizona State University, USA

Technical Program Committee

Nuno Correia   New University of Lisbon, Portugal

Publication Chair

Maria Pia Fanti   Politecnico di Bari, Italy

Publicity Chair

Walter Ukovich   University of Trieste, Italy

Local Chair

Chrysostomos D. Stylios   Technological Educational Institute of Epirus, Greece

Web Chair

Fotios Vartziotis   Technological Educational Institute of Epirus, Greece

Industry Track Chair

Spyridon Louvros   Technological Educational Institute of Messolonghi, Greece

Special Sessions Chair

Tiziana Catarci   University of Rome La Sapienza, Italy

Local Chair

Chrysostomos D. Stylios   Technological Educational Institute of Epirus,
                                 Greece

Web Chair

Fotios Vartziotis   Technological Educational Institute of Epirus,
                                 Greece

Conference Coordinator

Elisa Mendini   European Alliance for Innovation, Italy

Table of Contents

Full Papers

An Audio-Visual Database for Post-war Architecture and the City in
Greece... 1
Stavros Alifragkis and George Papakonstantinou

Game Design for Pre-screening Patients with Mental Health
Complications Using ICT Tools.................................... 16
Vibhuti Bagga, Kanav Kahol, and Sushil Chandra

Pervasiveness in Real-World Educational Games: A Case of Lego
Mindstorms and M.I.T App Inventor 23
Nikos Kalakos and Agis Papantoniou

Building Interactive Books Using EPUB and HTML5................. 31
Dimitris Gavrilis, Stavros Angelis, and Ioannis Tsoulos

Effects of Exercise in Diabetic Rats Using Continuous Wavelet
Transform 41
*Dimitrios G. Tsalikakis, Ioannis Nakos, Alexandros T. Tzallas,
Evagelos Karvounis, and Markos Tsipouras*

Managing Children's Asthma with a Low Cost Web-Enabled
Multifunctional Device 50
*Ioannis Smanis, George Poursanidis, Pantelis Angelidis,
Alexandros T. Tzallas, and Dimitrios Tsalikakis*

Integration of eHealth Service in IPv6 Vehicular Networks 65
*Sofiane Imadali, Athanasia Karanasiou, Alexandru Petrescu,
Ioannis Sifniadis, Eleftheria Vellidou, and Pantelis Angelidis*

Multimedia Chair Design for Improving the Experience of Hospital
Stay for Children with Cancer: The Escape......................... 81
Wout Kregting and Wei Chen

Devices and Wireless Interface Control in Vehicular Communications:
An Autonomous Approach 91
Michelle Wetterwald and Christian Bonnet

A 3.4-GHz Double Patch Pike-Shape Antenna for Wireless
Applications... 104
Constantinos T. Angelis, Eirini Tsiakalou, and Christos Koliopanos

Mobile Widget Technology as a Solution for Smart User Interaction 113
   Miroslav Behan and Ondrej Krejcar

Ambient Systems for the Environmental Monitoring: Characteristic
Examples at Different Spatial Scales................................ 123
   Stavros Kolios and Chrysostomos Stylios

Author Index.. 131

An Audio-Visual Database for Post-war Architecture and the City in Greece

Stavros Alifragkis[*] and George Papakonstantinou[**]

Laboratory of Environmental Communication & Audiovisual Documentation (LECAD),
Department of Architecture, School of Engineering, University of Thessaly
Pedion Areos, 38334 Volos, Greece
stavros.alifragkis@cantab.net, gpapakon@arch.uth.gr

Abstract. This paper reconsiders the notion of the archive in the context of a multimedia database for the city. It investigates the aesthetic and ideological constitution of the archive as a list, examines the nature of the urban historical evidence that is being transcribed into the conceptual setting of the database and, finally, experiments with the database as a storytelling mechanism that allows for multiple narrations about the city. A pilot, proof-of-concept interactive production experiments with an audiovisual database, initially comprising Greek newsreels and documentaries. This web-based prototype functions as the touchstone against which our main research questions are raised. The conceptual and production framework, outlined in this paper, represents work in progress conducted at the Laboratory of Environmental Communication and Audiovisual Documentation (LECAD) of the Department of Architecture, University of Thessaly. The project is generously funded by the Research Committee of the University of Thessaly and Thales Research Support Program.

Keywords: Database, List, Architecture, City, Cinema, Interactive, Metadata, Vocabularies.

1 Introduction

This paper readdresses the concept of the archive with reference to the representation of architecture and the city via the moving image. Here, some initial results from on-going research conducted at LECAD, Department of Architecture, University of Thessaly will be presented in brief. The project is generously funded by the Research Committee of the University of Thessaly and Thales Research Support Program. Using as a point of departure Lev Manovich and Umberto Eco's seminal work on the database and the list respectively, this research examines how our understanding of the city and its architecture can be shaped using the moving image as our primary resource. For this purpose, the project involves the setting up of an on-line multimedia

---

[*] Dr. Stavros Alifragkis is Post-doctoral Research Associate at LECAD, Department of Architecture, School of Engineering, University of Thessaly.
[**] George Papakonstantinou is Associate Professor at the Department of Architecture, School of Engineering, University of Thessaly.

C.T. Angelis, D. Fotiadis, and A.T. Tzallas (Eds.): AMBI-SYS 2013, LNICST 118, pp. 1–15, 2013.

database with existing footage, sourced from Greek newsreels, documentaries and family footage by individual contributors. Initially, the pilot prototype will be using archival material from the collections of the Hellenic National Audiovisual Archive from the 1950s and 1960s, when the Greek urban landscape experienced an unprecedented growth of construction activity. This entails handling approximately 250 newsreels that depict daily life, social events and state ceremonies in Athens and other Greek cities. Gradually, the audio-visual database will expand to include both Greek documentaries and more recent moving image works. Efforts will be made to enrich the database with complementary material from private collections that narrate the informal history of the city. The paper discusses the conceptual framework for setting up the project –compiling the audio-visual database and annotating with metadata the media files– and the digital tools utilized in the project.

2   Cinema and the City: Theoretical Framework

According to French philosopher, cultural theorist and urbanist Paul Virilio, early in the 20th century, perceptive faith –founded in the Middle Ages– began to lose ground over faith in the technical sightline. This crisis brought about the automation of perception and the production of synthetic vision afforded by technological advancement [1]. Virilio's 'eyeless vision' –the act of substituting the 'ideal alignment of the look' along an imaginary axis for a line of aim that 'appears thoroughly objective'– describes a great semantic loss in the history of perceptual faith [2]. No one managed to encapsulate this visual paradigm shift more comprehensively than the Soviet film-director Dziga Vertov (1896-1954). In Vertov's movie *The Man with the Movie Camera* (tMwtMC) [3] –originally intended to coincide with the tenth anniversary of the October Revolution– shots of the movie-camera and the machinegun are used interchangeably on several occasions. Vertov was determined that the human eye was not equipped to record the complexity, the multiplicity and the simultaneity of contemporary life [4]. Therefore, he sought to obtain unobstructed, unmediated and unbiased views of urban life via the omnipotent and omnipresent technologically advanced eye of the movie-camera, which always assumes an ideal point of view [5]. Montaged sequences with shots of the human eye, the camera lens and, finally, their visual overlap have become iconic of Vertov's theoretical package about cinema and particularly the act of catching 'life unawares' or, as film-historian Yuri Tsivian maintains, life 'off-guard.'[1] Vertov's anthropological laboratory was the Soviet city. His films constitute cinematic rhetorical arguments [8] that propagandize the link between the city and the countryside, between the peasantry and the proletariat [9]. In tMwtMC in particular, shots depicting the electrification of the USSR counterpoint dialectically shots portraying daily activities in no less than three major Soviet cities. These creative filmic reconstructions of the city suggest a wider understanding of the urban phenomena and their complexity, which is on par with some of the most contemporary urban theories [10]. Hence, the study of the celluloid metropolis not only enables alternative historical narratives about the urban form but also delivers

---

[1] The human eye/movie-camera superimposition is first introduced in Man Ray's experimental film entitled *Emak Bakia* [6]. The theme of the movie-camera and the cameraman is addressed in Sedgwick and Keaton's movie *The Cameraman* [7].

powerful heuristic devices for theorizing the city and imagining potential futures for the urban landscape.

Vertov's screen language epitomizes the formal and stylistic characteristics of a film genre that is generically referred to as 'city symphonies' or 'city films.' These are moving image works that encapsulate the dynamics of the modern metropolis by portraying a multitude of daily activities in the city and arranging them along a dawn-to-dusk narrative arc [11]. 'City symphonies' are characterized by certain formal features that distinguish them from other film genres. Indicatively, the main narrative mechanism that drives the story of a 'city film' forward is not based on human leads (protagonists, main characters, etc.), scripted dialogue and causally linked sequences and scenes, which have been associated with narrative cinema and classical Hollywood style in particular. Rather, the rhetorical ordering of brief vignettes on different urban themes –what could be construed as a visual argument for/against the city– dictates the episodic, fractal-like structure of many 'city films.' Furthermore, each brief, montaged vignette consists of shots depicting 'life unawares' in the city. Their succession in the narrative flow is regulated by complex editing rules that elicit analogies in the form and/or content between consecutive sequences and even shots. Finally, urban life is presented in documentary style, even though 'city films' do not constitute documentaries in the traditional sense [12]. 'City symphonies' were particularly popular in the 1920s and 1930s, however, their storytelling mechanism is still very much in use today, in the form of music videos, experimental moving image works, documentaries and brief montage intervals in fiction films.[2] The reconstruction of the image of the urban landscape in film is not exhausted in the study of 'city films.' The examination of other film genres, such as the film noir, has contributed greatly to our understanding of both the urban form and how it is perceived by everyday people. Nevertheless, the rigorous analysis and interpretation of the reconstructed celluloid city in classic 'city symphonies' from the 1930s, such as Ruttmann's *Berlin: Symphony of a Great City* [15] or Vigo's *On the Subject of Nice* [16], sharpen the conceptual and digital tools utilized in our investigation of the city in cinema.

The aim of our research project is to compile a multimedia database consisting of time-based media with a view to broadening our understanding of the Greek city and its architecture and to examining how societies perceived the urban landscape in the course of the second half of the 20th century. Moreover, the proposed proof-of-concept production intends to enable the potential user to navigate the database via a user-friendly, web-based interface. A set of project-specific options for interaction will enable the potential user to compile sequences of moving images on the fly, with media sourced from different content providers (newsreels, documentaries, family footage, etc.). The annotated with metadata media files of the audio-visual database will be thus reconfigured according to the rules that regulate the narrative structure of 'city symphonies' and Vertov's tMwtMC in particular. This approach was first introduced in a previous interactive moving image project by Alifragkis and Penz, *Cambridge City Symphony* [17].[3]

---

[2] Strand and Sheeler's *Manhatta* [13] constitutes one of the first 'city films' and Glawogger's *Megacities* [14] one of the latest.

[3] For additional information on the project refer to: Alifragkis, S., Penz, F. & Williams, D. 2006 [18].

Content-wise, it is crucial to determine early on what type of footage may be deemed relevant to our purposes. Protests, carnivals and festivals, promotional events, religious processions, outdoors performances, celebrations, riots, protests, art events and happenings, political rallies and official, State ceremonies describe only a fraction of the breadth and wealth of social events that take place in the city. Whether in the epicenter or as distant backgrounds of cinematic –fictional or documentary– narratives, these phenomena have been documented extensively by the camera-lens and function today as valuable resources for the urban historian and theoretician. Our project reserves a special place for media that captures unplanned, temporary and unconventional uses of the public space of the city –streets, squares, parks, public buildings, etc.– and enables an alternative historical narrative about the development of the urban form. We wish to construct a moving-image record of the landscape of the Greek metropolis, where marginal urban phenomena take center stage in the representation of daily city life on the screen. These often manifest themselves in the form of unorthodox and imaginative activities organized by grassroots urban social movements, who act locally in response to global socio-political stimuli [19]. Reclaiming disused or misused urban spaces and introducing alternative urban functions that promote high quality recreation over consumption constitutes fundamental issues that shape the current agenda on the future of the city. Media files sourced from newsreels and documentary films or personal raw footage will form a diverse pool of valuable moving image assets for the documentation and examination of the way public spaces in the city are weaved into the fabric of social life diachronically.

3   Media Annotation with Spatial Metadata

The initial stage of the project involves reviewing the results of similar, successfully completed projects and exploring the possibility of collaborating with research teams in Greece and abroad on the development of a common theoretical framework for discussing the urban form in film. An instance of the former, reviewing similar projects, is the AHRC-funded project entitled 'City in Film: Liverpool's Urban Landscape and the Moving Image' (2006-8), ran jointly by the School of Architecture and the Department of Communication and Media of the University of Liverpool [20]. The research team compiled a list of moving image files depicting the city of Liverpool, which were collated from a wide range of sources. The catalogue is publicly available on-line and users can search the collection using keywords such as: date, duration, genre, director/production credits, format (35mm, 16mm, 9.5mm, VHS, etc.), color/b&w, general synopsis, name and contact details of the archive holder or collector and viewing information, or:

'a list of locations and buildings; the architectural and urban space represented (e.g. public buildings and spaces, commercial and industrial areas, sites of leisure and recreation, education, health, religion, etc.); and the spatial use or function of the various spaces (e.g. festivals and parades, transit and mobility, everyday life, commercial, leisure, contested and political spaces, etc.)'[4] [24]

---

[4] For additional information on the project refer to Roberts & Koeck 2007:84-93 [21]; Hallam 2007:272-284 [22]; Roberts & Koeck 2007:7-11 [23].

Sadly, viewing the media files referenced in the list is currently unavailable. An instance of the latter, seeking collaborations, is the recently launched, AHRC-funded, collaborative project between the School of Architecture of the University of Liverpool and the Department of Architecture of the University of Cambridge entitled 'Cinematic Geographies of Battersea: Urban Interface & Site-Specific Spatial Knowledge' (2012-3) [25]. The research team has coined the term 'cinematic urban archaeology' to describe a systematic method of revisiting the city's recent past by carefully unveiling successive layers of celluloid reconstructions of the urban tissue. The aim of the project is to compile a database of relevant media files about Battersea, collated from official and unofficial –amateur filmmakers– sources. Furthermore, the team plans a series of 'urban interventions' that involve the use of cutting-edge information and communications technology and the digital media in order to augment the way people experience the city in their everyday lives. This will involve the recording and the subsequent retrieval of personal memories about specific sites by individual contributors. In this respect, asides enriching people's knowledge about Battersea's past, the project aims to reconstruct the area's unofficial history through oral testimonies. Likewise, LECAD will draw from relevant literature and experience with similar projects in order to address what appear to be two main research questions: a. how to describe the content of media files with reference to architecture and the city (media annotation); and b. how to navigate the database in a way that is both instructive and meaningful with reference to the reconstruction of the image of the city and the spatial mapping of digital data (media recycling). Media annotation is tackled in this section, while media recycling is discussed in the following part of our paper.

Umberto Eco draws our attention to the fact that both primitive and modern societies tend to resort to definitions that involve listing the properties of a substance rather than providing an account that signifies its essence. In other words, listing properties amounts to an enumeration of characteristics or inherent qualities and does not specify the 'what it is' of a substance. These lists, according to Aristotle, are essentially non-finite and, to a certain extent, arbitrary or accidental. Nevertheless, in everyday life, defining substances by listing their properties communicates more effectively data about our world, especially from the perspective of empirical thinking [26]. Therefore, researching the cinematic city could very well boil down to a list of accidental properties that serve the purpose of describing in detail –not exhaustively though– the visual and conceptual attributes of the city on the screen. This list of criteria could provide the much needed common denominator and provide justification for the compilation of a database –a diverse pool of media files– comprising footage that might appear to be otherwise unrelated to the untrained eye of the non-expert. In this early phase of our project, we experimented with a limited number of media resources –moving image clips containing single shots and/or brief sequences of shots– originating from three main sources: a. newsreels and documentaries from the Hellenic National Audiovisual Archive [27], b. documentaries and fiction films from the Greek Film Archive Foundation [28], and, most importantly, c. family videos, personal footage or amateur films submitted by

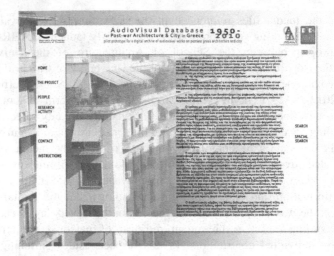

Fig. 1. The index page of the project's website

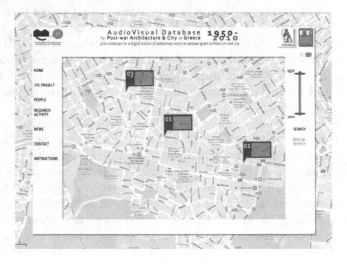

Fig. 2. Spatial mapping of metadata. Database assets are analyzed in scenes, sequences and shots. Subsequently, each element is pinpointed on the map by using its geographical location.

individuals to the official website of the project, which is currently under construction [29]. Essentially, this pilot, proof-of-concept production will attest which categories of spatial properties or urban features are most suited to the study of the city in film. These categories exist in the form of coded descriptive information pertaining to individual media files: database assets annotated with descriptive, structural and administrative metadata [30].

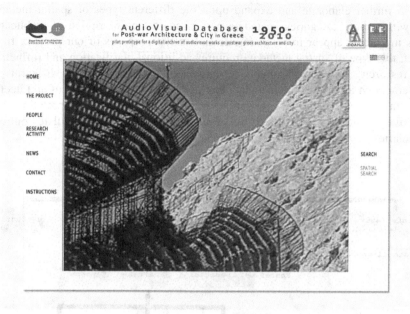

Fig. 3. Previewing window. Here, potential interactors may watch user-generated sequences of database items based on a set of finite options for navigating the audio-visual database.

Structural and administrative metadata have no particular bearing to the description of qualities that pertain to the reconstruction of the image of the city on the canvas of the screen. Conversely, descriptive metadata –or resource discovery metadata– is particularly relevant to our project, as it enables the potential user to identify, locate and retrieve relevant media files, by means of a finite set of categories. The categories introduced here foreground particular types of spatial information and attempt to highlight aspects of content that refer to specific urban features, such as the ones previously described in brief. Drawing from experience with earlier projects that utilized 'city symphonies' as raw material for studying the osmosis between the city and cinema (e.g. *Cambridge City Symphony*), we devised a set of limited criteria for the annotation of all media files with descriptive metadata [31]. Therefore, descriptive metadata can be further analyzed in three major categories: thematic metadata, spatial metadata and temporal metadata. Thematic metadata pertain to the description of the theme of a particular media file. As far as our research is concerned, themes are gleaned from relevant literature on urban planning as discussed below. Spatial metadata pertain to the description of filmic space. Finally, temporal metadata may refer to the date a media file was created but mostly to the era it depicts. Naturally, this research shows a special interest in the analysis and creative use of spatial metadata in particular. Here, we rely heavily on French film-director Eric Rohmer's study of space in cinema, as discussed in his 1972 work, first published in 1977, entitled *L' Organisation de l' Espace dans le Faust de Murnau* [32]. Hence, we utilize Rohmer's categories (pictorial space, architectural space and filmic space) in order to further elaborate and expand upon the different types of spatial metadata. Even within these categories, metadata pertaining to the description of architectural spaces in cinema appear to be more relevant to the purposes of our project. In this respect, this type of spatial metadata requires additional clarification and refinement. Our research introduces three subcategories, which tackle different but complementing aspects of the metadata that pertain to the description of architectural spaces in cinema: spatial categorisation, location, and spatial interpretation. Each respective subcategory is populated by a finite set of criteria that formulate controlled vocabularies.

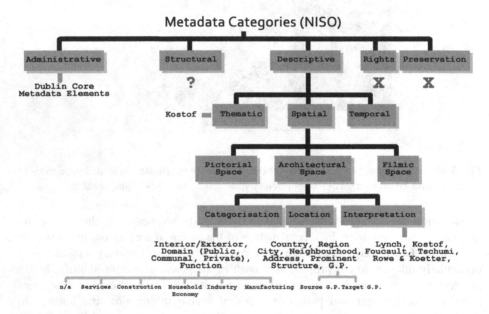

Fig. 4. *Metadata Categories.* Proposed analysis of *Descriptive Metadata* with a special focus on unearthing spatial features.

Vocabularies are introduced from existing literature on urban theory and history, with minor modifications where appropriate. Indicatively, one may examine the possibility of adopting urban themes from the widely discussed and much referenced work of architectural historian Spiro Kostof [33] [34]. Logging information about urban elements –the street, the square, the park, the natural limits, etc.– for each individual shot or sequence of shots could provide a loose narrative framework for the exploration of our diverse database.[5] The Greek Film Centre used to offer basic services in this direction, when the digitization of its limited collection was concluded in 2008 [35].[6] Currently, there is a call for offers for the design of a new on-line tool

---

[5] This line of inquiry is rather similar to the one the Liverpool-based research group pursued in 2008.

[6] The link is not active anymore.

for navigating the database with the use of descriptive metadata.[7] This straightforward approach provides a broadly accepted method for understanding and appreciating different urban, spatial categories. It remains to be seen whether it can trigger a more imaginative reshuffling of the assets in the database, hence the heuristic value of our pilot production. Our project seeks to explore alternative ways of exploiting the storytelling potentiality of visual or conceptual cues.embedded in our database items. One such way could be based on the creative reworking of Kevin Lynch's classic study on place legibility [36] –the creation of mental maps that illustrate very eloquently how city dwellers perceive the urban fabric– and the implementation of his set of unique urban elements –paths, edges, districts, nodes, and landmarks– for the annotation of the moving image assets of our database [37]. The latter may be supplemented with additional categories originating from the works of city theorists Colin Rowe and Fred Koetter's *Collage City* [38] and architect and theorist Bernard Tschumi's *Event Cities* [39]. The abovementioned studies are hardly complementary to each other. However, they represent significant shifts in the way specialists perceive the development and imagine the future of cities. In this respect, it would be interesting to see to what extent logging data about a wide range of urban features can sustain a more creative reshuffling of the database assets. The process of selecting a suitable framework of urban theory with a corresponding finite set of categories and subcategories and a hierarchical structure outlining their relations will be presented in detail in a future publication, as it falls slightly outside the scope of this paper.

Naturally, this research involves reviewing existing digital tools for the annotation of database assets, that is, logging descriptive metadata and experimenting with their storytelling potentialities. Currently, the all-pervasive spread of digital technologies offers a wide range of software that assists various types of research for different research phases in the arts and humanities.[8] Furthermore, several software packages have been designed for the purpose of logging, computing and visualizing aspects of film style, based on the annotation of individual shots. In 2005, the collaboration between film historian Yuri Tsivian and computer scientist Gunars Civjans resulted in the production of 'CineMetrics,' a 'movie measurement and study tool database' that enables the logging and processing of stylistic metadata [41]. The software uses two modes, 'simple' and 'advanced.' 'Simple' mode allows the user to manually log shots while watching the movie with the play-back software of her/his choice. Here one can calculate the number of shots, shot duration and the Average Shot Length. 'Advanced' mode functions in a similar way, but allows for the logging of different types of metadata via eight user-customized buttons. Basic statistical processing is readily available, but more advanced handling of the metadata –including the visualization of the statistical processing– is possible only when one submits the results to the online database. Based on Tsivian and Civjans' 'CineMetrics,' 'Shot Logger' –developed at the Department of Telecommunication & Film of the

---

[7] For additional information on the forthcoming project for a digital archive please refer to: http://www.gfc.gr/index.php?option=com_content&task=view&id=12 83&Itemid=118&lang=en [last accessed: 07/05/12].

[8] For the various tools offered today refer to: Digital tools: Arts-Humanities.Net: Guide to Digital Humanities & Arts [40].

University of Alabama by Professor Jeremy Butler– allows the user to manually capture and log shots and, in addition to other software, generate screen-shots and attach them to the statistical data [42]. In 2007, the Vienna-based research group entitled 'Digital Formalism' –a collaboration between the Department of Theatre, Film and Media Studies of the University of Vienna, the Austrian Film Museum, and the Interactive Media Systems Group of the Vienna University of Technology– embarked on an ambitious project that involved, among other tasks, performing a computer-aided analysis of Vertov's work [43].[9] The group utilized 'Anvil' for the annotation of Vertov's tMwtMC [45]. This rather sophisticated piece of software, designed and programmed by Michael Kipp –Professor for interactive media at the University of Applied Sciences in Augsburg, Germany– is a free moving-image annotation tool that offers 'hierarchical multi-layered annotation driven by user-defined schemes.' 'Deconstructor' was introduced in 2002 by filmmaker and Adjunct Professor at the Film Division of the School of the Arts at Columbia University Larry Engel as 'a constructivist approach to learning about film' [46].[10] 'Deconstructor' accommodated: a. scene and shot preview and detection in 'storyboard' mode (duration, in point, out point); b. annotation of shots in 'databoard' mode (graphic arrangement, shot type, shot angle, shot perspective, camera movement, camera movement type, camera movement value, subject movement, subject movement direction, subject movement to/from camera, subject movement zoom strength, entrance and exit); and c. generation of graphs based on the statistical analysis of the accumulated metadata. This on-line tool is no longer available. One of the most practical on-line tools for logging metadata is the aptly called 'Vertov,' a media annotating plug-in for 'Zotero,' which is an on-line tool for managing resources [48]. With 'Vertov' one could mark in and out points on the timeline of locally-stored media files and annotate individual shots or sequences. There were no predefined categories, only plain text boxes. Vertov could generate screen-shots but it could not process the metadata statistically. Currently, the plug-in is inactive. 'ImagePlot' by Lev Manovich, Professor of Visual Arts, University of California, San Diego, is 'a free software tool that visualizes collections of images and video of any size' [49]. It has proven to be very reliable and grants the user a great degree of freedom that enables extremely diverse and imaginative visual representations of the annotated metadata, with artistic merit in their own right. Less reliable freeware is available on-line. These vary in sophistication, functionality, and accuracy. Some boast automatic detection of shots or movement within the shot (e.g. surveillance software). These are extremely unreliable, especially with low quality, b&w footage. Our research experiments with the functionalities offered by 'Anvil.'

4   Media Recycling: Database Narrative and the City

Eco argues that a list is much more than a compilation of items bound together by certain attributes, shared in common under the pretext of a mutual denominator. The

---

[9] For additional information on the project refer to: Kropf et al. 2009:117-132 [44].
[10] For additional information on the software refer to: Sosulski et al. 2004 [47].

list is a powerful art form with immense storytelling potentiality. British film-director and digital media artist Peter Greenaway has been experimenting with the list as a storytelling mechanism ever since his first feature-length movie entitled *The Falls* [50]. Greenaway uses linear narratives as a stepping stone for his multi-focal cinematic narrations, which transcend the expressive confines of film and spill over to neighboring artistic fields such as opera, art exhibitions, happenings and art-books [51]. His moving image experiments illustrate what Manovich terms 'competing imaginations' in new media cultures: database and narrative [52]. Manovich suggests that sequential, cause-and-effect, single or multiple storyline trajectories (narrative threads) and unstructured, non-hierarchical collections of items (databases) take on different statuses as far as contemporary computer culture is concerned. Naturally, he prefers the latter over the former, as database narratives put into effective use functionalities afforded by current technological advances with computer software.

Databases may consist of unstructured media files but the navigation of the database can rely heavily on complex sets of predefined rules described by the author, which can be manipulated –to a certain extent– by the user. Manovich, commenting on his multimedia interactive production entitled *Soft Cinema*, notes that:

> '[t]he DVD was designed and programmed so that there is no single version of any of the films. All the elements –including screen layout, the visuals and their combination, the music, the narrative, and the length– are subject to change every time the film is viewed.' [53]

Marsha Kinder attempts to provide the following working definition for database narratives:

> 'Database narratives refers to narratives whose structure exposes or thematizes the dual processes of selection and combination that lie at the heart of all stories and that are crucial to language: the selection of particular data [...] from a series of databases or paradigms, which are then combined to generate specific tales.' [54]

Our aim is to generate multiple itineraries across the database assets by developing a 'selection of particular data' –transcribing and modifying existing spatial categories from relevant literature and/or devising new– that pertains to the creative reconsideration of aspects of urban form. Utilizing software for the manual and automated annotation of our database items –with descriptive metadata about the city and its architecture– is expected to enable a more creative –even artistic– use of the archive and result in a better understanding of its valuable contents. This aspect of the project is referred to as media recycling and describes an extremely potent and current area of artistic endeavor. The practice of using and reusing footage in different storytelling frameworks is fairly common, especially with particular types of production (newsreels, documentaries, experimental movies, music videos, advertisements). In the 1920's, Vertov, for example, used to recycle his own material –even footage captured by others– into new productions, due to the scarcity of raw materials and time constraints. However, a practice that was born out of necessity soon became a matter of aesthetic choice.[11] In this context, retrieving, ordering

---

[11] See for example Sfikas' *Metropolises* [55] or Shub's *The Fall of the Romanov Dynasty* [56].

sequentially and previewing database items that meet specific criteria –i.e. shots, sequences and/or scenes that address Lynch's notion of the 'edge' or render visually what Tschumi describes as an 'event'– from a much larger pool of media files, could reveal new ways of working with digital, moving image archives. The juxtaposition of media files from diverse sources dictated by a specific set of montage rules might bring forth otherwise unattained analogies or contradictions between the database assets.

5   Concluding Remarks

Evidently, the final deliverable of this project will be a user-friendly, web-based interactive production, where potential users –both researchers and the general public– will be able to locate, configure on the fly and preview a succession of shots that have been sourced from different narratological contexts (documentaries, fiction films, newsreels, family videos). Their ordering will be based on user-defined, project-specific spatial categories. Ideally, the production will serve as a digital workspace, where people can upload amateur films or home videos and contribute to the logging of basic or more advanced descriptive metadata. The technology for something like this already exists. In 2007, the American electronic media artist Perry Bard initiated a participatory reworking of Vertov's tMwtMC over the internet. She developed a web-based application where individual users can:

> '[i]nterpret Vertov and upload [...] footage to [the] site to become part of the database. [They] can contribute an entire scene or a shot or multiple shots from different scenes. [...] Every day a new version of the film is compiled from shots uploaded to the site.' [57]

Bard's project is particularly relevant to our research as it manages to successfully combine the analysis and interpretation of an existing moving image work on the one hand and innovative and artistic experimentation with visual communication on the other. Similarly, our proposed web-based application will enable the potential user to revisit and reassess the city's recent past via the creative reconfiguration its image on film. Hopefully, this visual retrospection of the urban form will generate a more wide-ranging discussion about the potential futures of the Greek city.

Acknowledgments. The authors wish to thank Mrs. Ifigenia Charatsi (laboratory staff at LECAD) and Mr. Giorgos Kalaouzis (computer engineer and laboratory teaching staff at LECAD) for their invaluable help in all phases of the research and production. Also, the authors wish to acknowledge and thank the Research Committee of the University of Thessaly for funding the initial phase of our study and the research project 'DEMUCIV, Designing the Museum of the City of Volos' (2012-2015) – funded by the Thales Research Support Program under the Greek Ministry of Education Lifelong Learning and Religion and the European Union– for funding the second and final stage of our research.

References

1. Virilio, P.: The Vision Machine, pp. 13, 16, 59–76. Indiana University Press, British Film Institute, London, Bloomington (1994)
2. Virilio, P.: War and Cinema: The Logistics of Perception, pp. 2–3. Verso, London (2000)
3. Vertov, D.: The Man with the Movie Camera [Film]. USSR, 68' (1929)
4. Vertov, D.: Kino-Eye: The Writings of Dziga Vertov, pp. 40–42. University of California Press, Berkeley (1984)
5. Heath, S.: Questions of Cinema, p. 32. Indiana University Press, Bloomington (1981)
6. Ray, M.: Emak Bakia [Film]. France, 18' (1927)
7. Sedgwick, E., Keaton, B.: The Cameraman [Film]. US, 69' (1928)
8. Bordwell, D., Thompson, K.: Film Art: An Introduction, pp. 102–141. McGraw-Hill, New York (1993)
9. Porter, R.: The City in Russian Literature: Images Past and Present. The Modern Language Review 94(2), 476 (1999)
10. Alifragkis, S., Penz, F.: Fragmented Utopias - Architecture, Literature and the Cinematic Image of the Ideal Socialist City of the Future: Dziga Vertov's Man with a Movie Camera. In: Harris, J., Williams, R.J. (eds.) Regenerating Culture and Society: Architecture, Art and Urban Style within the Global Politics of City-Branding, pp. 117–141. Liverpool University Press & Tate Liverpool, Liverpool (2011)
11. Penz, F.: Architecture and the Screen from Photography to Synthetic Imaging - Capturing and Building Space, Time and Motion. In: Thomas, M., Penz, F. (eds.) Architecture of Illusion: From Motion Pictures to Navigable Interactive Environments, pp. 135–164. Intellect, Bristol (2003)
12. Alifragkis, S.: City Symphonies - Restructuring the Urban Landscape: Dziga Vertov's Man with the Movie Camera and the City of the Future [PhD Thesis]. Department of Architecture, University of Cambridge, Cambridge (2010)
13. Strand, P., Sheeler, C.: Manhatta [Film]. US, 11' (1921)
14. Glawogger, M.: Megacities [Film]. Austria, Switzerland, 90' (1998)
15. Ruttmann, W.: Berlin: Symphony of a Great City [Berlin: Die Sinfonie der Großtadt] [Film]. Germany, 65' (1927)
16. Vigo, J.: On the Subject of Nice [À Propos de Nice] [Film]. France, 25' (1930)
17. Cambridge City Symphony, http://expressivespace.org/research-NM2-p3.html
18. Alifragkis, S., Penz, F., Williams, D.: D3.3: An Introduction to NM2 Production Cambridge City Symphony [Project Report]. New Media for the New Millennium, Cambridge, Ipswich (2006)
19. Castells, M.: The City and the Grassroots. University of California Press, Berkeley (1983)
20. City in Film: Liverpool's Urban Landscape and the Moving Image,
http://www.arts-humanities.net/projects/
city_film_liverpools_urban_landscape_moving_image
21. Roberts, L., Koeck, R.: The Archive City: Reading Liverpool's Urban Landscape through Film. In: Grunenberg, C., Knifton, R. (eds.) Centre of the Creative Universe: Liverpool and the Avant-Garde, pp. 84–93. Liverpool University Press, Liverpool (2007)
22. Hallam, J.: Mapping City Space: Independent Filmmakers as Urban Gazetteers. Journal of British Cinema and Television 4(2), 272–284 (2007)
23. Roberts, L., Koeck, R.: Liverpool in Film: Mapping the Past in the Present. Liverpool School of Architecture Journal 1, 7–11 (2007)

24. Mapping the City in Film: A Geo-historical Analysis, http://www.liv.ac.uk/lsa/cityinfilm/
25. Cinematic Geographies of Battersea, http://cinematicbattersea.blogspot.co.uk/ and http://www.expressivespace.org/battersea.html
26. Eco, U.: The Infinity of Lists, pp. 217–221. Rizzoli, New York (2009)
27. Hellenic National Audiovisual Archive, http://mam.avarchive.gr/portal/
28. Greek Film Archive Foundation, http://www.tainiothiki.gr/v2/lang_en/index/index/
29. An Audio-visual Database for Post-war Architecture and the City in Greece, http://www.arch.uth.gr/sites/arch-city-avdb
30. Wilson, A., et al.: Digital Moving Images and Sound Archiving Study, pp. 67–90. Arts and Humanities Data Service, London (2006)
31. Alifragkis, S., Penz, F.: Spatial Dialectics: Montage and Spatially Organised Narrative in Stories without Human Leads. Digital Creativity 17(4), 221–233 (2006)
32. Rohmer, É.: L' Organisation de l' Espace dans le Faust de Murnau. Cahiers du Cinéma, Paris (2000)
33. Kostof, S.: The City Assembled: Elements of Urban Form through History. Thames & Hudson, New York (2005)
34. Kostof, S.: The City Shaped: Urban Patterns and Meanings Through History. Thames & Hudson, New York (1999)
35. Greek Film Centre: Digital Archive, http://www.gfcdigital.gr/gfc/index.html
36. Lynch, K.: The Image of the City. Massachusetts Institute of Technology, Cambridge (1960)
37. Alifragkis, S., et al.: Production Report: Cambridge City Symphony [Project Report]. New Media - New Millennium, Cambridge (2006)
38. Rowe, C., Koetter, F.: Collage City. Massachusetts Institute of Technology, Cambridge (1978)
39. Tschumi, B.: Event Cities. Massachusetts Institute of Technology, Cambridge (1994)
40. Digital tools: Arts-Humanities.Net: Guide to Digital Humanities & Arts, \ http://www.arts-humanities.net/
41. Cinemetrics, http://www.cinemetrics.lv/index.php
42. Shot Logger, http://shotlogger.org/index.php
43. Digital Formalism, http://www.isis.tuwien.ac.at/node/4850
44. Kropf, V., et al.: First Steps Towards Digital Formalism: The Vienna Vertov Collection. In: Ross, M., et al. (eds.) Digital Tools in Media Studies: Analysis and Research: An Overview, pp. 117–132. Transcript Verlag, Bielefeld (2009)
45. Anvil, http://www.anvil-software.de/
46. Deconstructor, http://ccnmtl.columbia.edu/projects/engel/deconstructor/index.html
47. Sosulski, A.K., et al.: The Deconstructor. Providing the Scaffolds for Students to Excerpt, Describe, Analyze, Interpret and Synthesize to Form New Understandings (2004), http://citeseerx.ist.psu.edu/viewdoc/summary?doi=10.1.1.116.668 (last accessed: September 01, 2012)
48. Centre for Oral History and Digital Storytelling, http://storytelling.concordia.ca/; Vertov: A Media Annotating Plugin for Zotero, http://digitalhistory.concordia.ca/vertov/

49. ImagePlot,
    http://lab.softwarestudies.com/p/imageplot.html#features1
50. Greenaway, P.: The Falls [Film]. UK, 195' (1980)
51. Greenaway, P.: 100 Objects to Represent the World: A Prop Opera. Thessaloniki International Film Festival, Thessaloniki (1998)
52. Manovich, L.: The Language of New Media, p. 233. Massachusetts Institute of Technology, Cambridge (2001)
53. Manovich, L., et al.: Soft Cinema: Navigating the Database [Interactive Production]. ZKM, Berlin (2002-2003)
54. Kinder, M.: Hot Spots, Avatars, and Narrative Fields Forever. Film Quarterly 55(4), 2–15 (2002)
55. Sfikas, K.: Metropolises [Film]. Greece (1975)
56. Shub, E.: The Fall of the Romanov Dynasty [Film]. USSR, 90' (1927)
57. Man with a Movie Camera – The Participatory Global Remake,
    http://dziga.perrybard.net/

Game Design for Pre-screening Patients with Mental Health Complications Using ICT Tools

Vibhuti Bagga[1], Kanav Kahol[1], and Sushil Chandra[2]

[1] Public Health Foundation of India
[2] Institute of Nuclear Medicine and Allied Sciences, Defence Research & Development Organization, India
{vibhuti.bagga,Kanav.kahol}@phfi.org, sushil.inmas@gmail.com

Abstract. Mental health disorders are significant contributors to the global burden of diseases. Conventional approach to mental health screening involves administration of specially designed questionnaires and tests by mental health professionals. In the current global scenario where adequate mental health professionals are not available, video-games can serve as an important aid for mental health screening. This paper discusses a framework for designing games for cognitive assessment and using the ubiquitous nature of computing to serve as a platform for mental health screening. Neuropsychological tests can be embedded within the game structure for cognitive assessment. To establish the viability of this concept a pilot study was carried out. A game was developed with an aim to assess the player's stress levels. Stress affects working memory and attention span. The prison game implements the Digit Span test for attention span and working memory assessment. The validity of such a game is demonstrated through an experiment. The results of the experiment analysis indicate that the short term stress experienced by the players can be successfully predicted based on the performance in the cognitive game.

Keywords: mental health, stress, video games, neurocognitive assessment, EEG, PCA.

1 Introduction

Mental health is an integral part of every individual's fitness. WHO defines Mental Health as not just the absence of mental disorder but as a state of well-being in which every individual realizes his or her own potential, can cope with the normal stresses of life, can work productively and fruitfully, and is able to make a contribution to her or his community. But despite being such an important aspect of health, mental health scenario has been in a dismal state for many decades the world over. The awareness about the prevalence of the mental/cognitive disorders and its treatment is negligible. It goes undiagnosed in most cases. About 76-85 % of people with severe mental disorders receive no treatment for their health problems in low and middle income countries while in high income countries the range is 35-50%.

Although there have not been many conclusive epidemiological studies, psychiatrists estimate that in India around 7 % of the population suffers from mental disorders. As per the WHO-AIMS report, in terms of resources, India has 0.25 beds

C.T. Angelis, D. Fotiadis, and A.T. Tzallas (Eds.): AMBI-SYS 2013, LNICST 118, pp. 16–22, 2013.

per 10,000 population (0.2 in mental hospital and 0.05 in general hospitals) while there are 0.2 psychiatrists per 1,00,000 people. The scene in rural areas is worse. Due to the social stigma associated with being mentally sick most of the people do not go to a psychiatrist or seek any medical help.

In such circumstances, ICT and video games offers a new approach towards bridging the gap between the need and available resources for mental health. The ubiquitous nature of computing technologies can be translated into a medium of affordable, easily and widely available tool for screening people for mental health problems by assessing their cognitive abilities. Besides making mental healthcare more accessible, pre-screening patients can effectively ease the load on existing infrastructure for mental health.

Gaming and cognitive assessment has been a subject of many studies. Games are affordable and can be scaled to large deployments as they are offered on commercial platforms and are robust. They are engaging and are designed for long term usage. Mental fitness is divided into its constituent components such as attention, long term memory, short term memory, intermodal coordination etc[1-2]. A game for cognitive assessment employs the foundations of neuropsychological testing. Neuropsychological assessment is an active research area in medicine where meticulously designed tests are employed to measure cognitive abilities of patients [3-7]. This is done primarily to evaluate abilities of patients with stroke, neural disorders and neural trauma. Based on these tests, several compendiums have been established that help evaluate baseline cognitive abilities of patients and the normative population. Lezak et al. have developed a list of several such tests.

For a game to serve as a more effective and efficient tool for assessment of desired cognitive skill-set, it needs to be designed such that the game events and the implicit cognitive elements are mapped, standardized and the game flow is able to adjust dynamically in response to the cognitive feedback. The proposed framework is shown in Figure1.

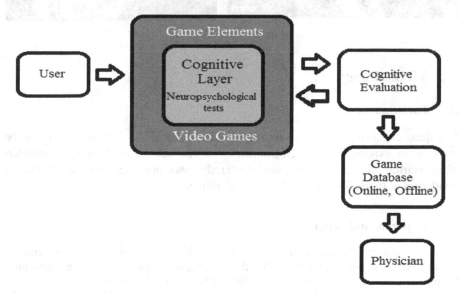

Fig. 1. Framework for designing games for cognitive assessment

The assessment results obtained through the game can be sent online to a physician specializing in mental health in case there are any indications of mental health impairment.

This paper introduces a prison themed game that has been developed based on the above discussed framework and has been designed with an aim to assess the player's level of stress. A number of different research studies have shown that stress impairs working memory formation [8], [10]. There are many neuropsychological tests that give a measure of working memory such as the digit span task, Sternberg item recognition task, n-back test etc. The digit span test [6] requires memorizing a sequence of numbers presented visually or through audio and recalling those numbers either immediately or after a time gap. The prison game represents an implementation of the test in gaming scenario where a player has to remember the sequence to accomplish certain action. Thus, stress levels of a person can be identified by assessing working memory and attention span through this game.

A pilot study was carried out to test the effectiveness of the prison game developed to assess stress levels. The following sections describe the methodology and results obtained.

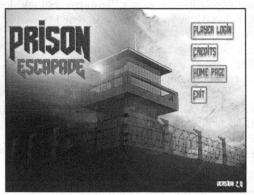 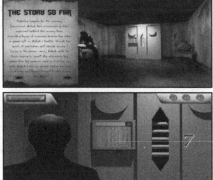

Fig. 2. Prison Game

2   Methodology

2.1   Participants

14 subjects engaged in different white collar jobs, aged 22-41 years volunteered to be a part of the experiment. Written informed consent was obtained from the subjects before starting the experiment and the study was approved by Public Health Foundation of India, Institutional Ethics Committee.

2.2   Experimental Setup

Game description: The prison game has been developed using the unity game engine. The story line revolves around a soldier that has been captured in the enemy territory. The player's task is to help in rescuing the soldier and bring him back to homeland. The first level opens in the high security prison cell where the soldier is confined. To unlock the cell door the player needs to enter the electronic key codes that the trapped soldier tries to reminisce. For each correct code the soldier gains health points and moves a step further in the rescue. Three incorrect codes set the prison alarms ringing and rescue mission fails. The profiles of each player were maintained in the game. An offline on-disk as well as an online server based record of the players' performance was also maintained.

Stress Assessment: a couple of stress questionnaires and self-reporting was used as direct measures of stress levels of the player. In self reporting the subjects were asked to rate the stress levels they experienced just before playing the game, an hour before gameplay, 1 day before gameplay and their average levels of stress, on a scale of 1-10.

Assessment of working memory and attention span: The game itself implements the neuropsychological test: digit span which gives a measure of working memory and attention span. However, to test and validate the implementation, another test known as the N-Back Test was used for direct assessment. The N-Back test requires the subject to report when a stimulus item (visual or auditory) presented serially is the same as an item 'N' steps back for the time at hand. For the 2-back condition if the sequence were 8-7-1-8-6-3-6, the subject would indicate his response verbally by saying 'yes' after the second 6. In this experiment, a 2-Back test was used with visual stimuli.

Physiological Correlates: During game play physiological data in the form of EEG (electroencephalography) was collected using the Emotive Epoc headset. The EEG headset allows data to be recorded from 14 scalp locations viz. AF3, F7, F3, FC5, T7, P7, O1, O2, P8, T8, FC6, F4, F8, AF4. The data was sampled at 128 Hz.

Protocol: After the informed consent forms were signed and collected, each subject was asked to fill the stress questionnaire and self-reporting questions. Then they were subjected to the N-Back test. Following this the subjects were required to play the prison game for a minimum of three sessions (~15-20 min). After the gameplay the subjects were debriefed. The EEG data was recorded during the entire game play.

3   Analysis

The different variables such as scores of the stress questionnaires and self-reporting, the number of correct numeric key codes entered to open the door of the prison cell, the length of the codes, the accuracy in the game, N-Back test scores, average time to respond in the N-back test etc., were subjected to statistical analysis. The variables were checked for correlation using SPSS. The following equation is used to calculate the Pearson's correlation coefficient:

$$r = \frac{\Sigma(x * y)}{N * \sigma x * \sigma y}$$

Where,

r = Karl pearson's co-efficient of correlation

x = mean deviation of X

y = mean deviation of Y

$$\sigma x = \text{standard deviation of X}$$
$$\sigma y = \text{standard deviation of Y}$$
$$N = \text{number of pairs of observation}$$

The EEG data epochs corresponding to different game events such as the time period when each numeric code was displayed on the screen, the response time of the user etc. were isolated. Each isolated epoch was filtered and divided into the 5 frequency bands viz. delta(0.5-4 Hz), theta(4-8 Hz), alpha(8-13 Hz), beta(13-30) and gamma(>30) using 6th order butterworth bandpass filters. This EEG data was then subjected to principal component analysis.

4   Results

The reported stress levels before playing the game were found to be negatively correlated with total number of attempts, accuracy in the game, maximum length of the numeric key codes in each game session and N-Back test scores. The scores of the questionnaires are positively correlated with the average levels of stress as reported. Table 1 shows the different variables and values of correlation coefficient.

The principal component analysis indicates that the immediate stress levels can be predicted with an accuracy of 87.5 % on the basis of the player's EEG during epochs corresponding to the time when the numeric key codes are displayed. This game event is a part of the implementation of the neuropsychological test digit span.

Table 1. Correlation analysis

		Pearsonian Correlation	Sig.(2-tailed)
TA	ISL	-0.614	0.02
AGP	ISL	-0.741	0.002
MLAvg	ISL	-0.615	0.019
N-Back Test Scores	ISL	-0.589	0.027
N-Back Test Scores	AGP	0.814	0.000
N-Back Test Scores	TA	0.795	0.001
N-Back Test Scores	MLAvg	0.863	0.000
SQAvg	AvgSL	0.653	0.011

ISL   = Reported Stress levels immediately before Gameplay
MLS1 = Max. length of numeric key codes in Session1
MLS2 = Max. length of numeric key codes in Session2
MLS3 = Max. length of numeric key codes in Session3
MLAvg = Average Maximum Length
SQAvg = Average Score in Stress Questionnaires
AvgSL = Average levels of stress experienced by the subject as reported
AGP   = Accuracy in Gameplay
TA   = Total Attempts

5   Conclusions

The focus of this analysis is to investigate the possibility of developing customized games for cognitive assessment based on the proposed framework. To fulfill this aim a prison game was developed to assess a player's stress levels. Significant co-relation was found between many of the analyzed variables.

Stress affects working memory and attention span. By assessing these cognitive components, the stress levels of a subject can be estimated. The scores of the N-Back test were positively correlated with game accuracy and average maximum code length. This validates the implementation of the digit span test in the cognitive game developed. The results of the analysis indicate that the short term stress experienced by the players can be predicted based on the performance in the game as well as the EEG signals of the player during game-play.

References

1. Lezak, M.D.: Neuropsychological assessment, 4th edn. Oxford University Press, Oxford (2004)
2. Kahol, K., Panchanathan, S.: Neurocognitively inspired haptic user interfaces. Springer Journal on Multimedia Tools and Applications 37(1), 15–38 (2007)
3. Gevins, A., Smith, M.E., Le, J.: High resolution evoked potential imaging of the cortical dynamics of human working memory. Electroencephalogr. Clin. Neurophysiol. 98(4), 327–348 (1996)
4. Klove, H.: Clinical Neuropsychology: The medical clinics of North America. Saunders, New York (1963)
5. Levendowski, D.J., Berka, C., Olmstead, R.E., Jarvik, M.: Correlations between EEG Indices of Alertness Measures of Performance and Self-Reported States while Operating a Driving Simulator. Paper Presented at: 29th Annual Meeting, Society for Neuroscience, Miami Beach, FL (1999)
6. Lezak, M.D., Howieson, D.B., Loring, D.: Neuropsychological Assessment. Oxford, New York (2004)
7. Westbrook, P., Berka, C., Levendowski, D.J.: Quantification of Alertness, Memory and Neurophysiological Changes in Sleep Apnea Patients Following Treatment with nCPAP. Sleep 27(A223) (2004)

8. Luethi, M., Meier, B., Sandi, C.: Stress effects on working memory, explicit memory & implicit memory for neutral and emotional stimuli in healthy men. Frontiers in Behavioral Neuroscience (2009)
9. Marin, M.F., Lord, C., Andrews, J., Juster, R.P., Sindi, S., Arsenault-Lapierre, G., Fiocco, A.J., Lupien, S.J.: Chronic stress, cognitive functioning and mental health. Neurobiology of Learning and Memory 96(4), 583–595 (2011)
10. Kuhlmann, S., Piel, M., Wolf, O.T.: Impaired memory retrieval after psychosocial stress in healthy young men. The Journal of Neuroscience, 2977–2982 (2005)

Pervasiveness in Real-World Educational Games: A Case of Lego Mindstorms and M.I.T App Inventor

Nikos Kalakos[1] and Agis Papantoniou[2]

[1] Fokida's Department of Secondary Education, Amfissa, Greece,
nikalakos@sch.gr
[2] National Technical University of Athens, School of Electrical & Computer Engineering,
Athens, Greece,
apapant@medialab.ntua.gr

Abstract. Without a doubt, children consider mobile phones to be something more than just a means of communication. It is, actually, an extension of themselves and an integral part of their lives. The unique relationship that they have developed with these devices, which has been reinforced with the launching of smartphones, could not be left unnoticed by the educational community as every successful educational activity does not exist without the motivation of students via a climate of enthusiasm and the constant providing of incentives. Games, digital or otherwise, at school fall under the same category. Their blending and the children's response to them are particularly interesting and, thus have triggered off the creation of a game, presented within the context of this paper. This game, designed for smartphones with android O.S, was developed through the M.I.T. App Inventor programming environment, which interacts with Lego Mindstorms robotic constructions.

Keywords: smartphones, educational robotics, digital games, M.I.T. App Inventor, digital game-based learning, educational programming environment.

1 Introduction

According to contemporary educational theories, the main goal of the educator today should be to establish a teamwork-research environment within which students, through appropriate activities, would be able to shape the new knowledge themselves. This is a procedure in which the educator acts as a facilitator and incorporates a series of processes such as searching and scanning the given information via multiple sources, evaluating the newly-acquired knowledge, experimenting, discovering, problem-solving and giving feedback. Dewey [1], for that matter, advocates that children's education should be based on their innate instincts for questioning, building, expression and communication. Experiential education plays a crucial role to the effectiveness of the above theories as far as the meaning and the practice of a methodology towards problem-solving are concerned as well as towards the existence of suitable motivation for their involvement in the educational activities.

C.T. Angelis, D. Fotiadis, and A.T. Tzallas (Eds.): AMBI-SYS 2013, LNICST 118, pp. 23–30, 2013.

Educational robotics and programming, not just as a school subject but as a theoretical method, are prerequisites for the realization of the first factor as it is evident through the widespread use of the programmed robotic kit of Lego Mindstorms NXT[1] in education, as well as of other educational programming applications, most popular of which are M.I.T. Scratch[2], Alice[3] and logo-environments, such as StarLogo[4].

On the other hand, key to the success of the second factor is the use of the children's special interests and activities. Taking into account that they are the "natives" of today's digital world [2], and considering the pertinent research [3][4] that testify for the intense drawing of the youth generally towards smartphones and especially towards mobile gaming, it is made clear why the educational community for the last few years has been focused on integrating digital games (Digital Game Based Learning) and mobile phones devices (Mobile Learning) into the educational process. Since the benefits for education that derive from the use of the above technologies are substantiated, it is interestingly challenging to search for methods and processes that would allow for their combining use under a united platform within the learning process. M.I.T. App Inventor[5] has made it possible for the development of the game which is presented in this paper, whose objective is to examine whether and to what extent the combination of Educational Robotics – Digital Games – Smartphones could add on to the enthusiasm, the motivation and the active participation of children in the learning process.

According to the above, the structure of the paper is as follows: In section 2, background information is presented concerning the tools and the methodology used for the development of the game. In section 3, the game is presented along with a discussion upon the results of its application in the Gravia Secondary School. Finally, in section 4, the authors of the paper conclude their research and propose further areas for improvement.

2   Tools and Methods

2.1   M.I.T. App Inventor

M.I.T. App Inventor is a new visual programming internet environment which allows for the creation of applications for smartphones with android operational system. This was presented by Google in 2010, and as of January 2012 M.I.T. has been in charge of its support and development. The commands are given through predetermined coloured tiles, which are connected just like the pieces of a puzzle to form command blocks activated upon realization of an event (event driven programming) (Fig.1).

---

[1] http://mindstorms.lego.com/en-us/Default.aspx
[2] http://scratch.mit.edu
[3] http://www.alice.org
[4] http://education.mit.edu/starlogo
[5] http://appinventor.mit.edu

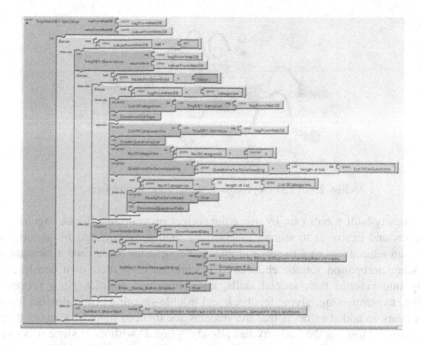

Fig. 1. App Inventor's Programming Environment

Thus, the chances for syntactic errors to occur are minimized as, like with the puzzle, the tiles have special incisions and projections that prevent the connection of tiles "non-syntactically connected". The development of the application's interface is a simple procedure which involves the placing of set components through drag n'drop on the screen of a virtual smartphone. It involves a wide range of possibilities like creating and processing local and remote Databases, using Bluetooth technology, supporting multiple screens and managing Lego Mindstorms robotic structures. Since it is still in beta edition, it is currently undergoing improvements and additions of new functions. The trial and error of the programs can be done either by connecting the mobile phone to the computer, or by using the installed emulator. The applications formed can run in all smartphones with an android system and can be intershared through Google Play.

This is an innovative tool, as its development environment allows for the formation of complex and demanding applications even by people with minimum experience and knowledge in programming in an easy, fast and, most importantly, entertaining way.

2.2   Lego Mindstorms NXT

Lego's educational robots have been around since 1998 and within a few years have succeeded in being a reference point for education. They involve a group of sensors, Lego bricks, motors, service mechanisms and other components which form constructions programmed through a microprocessor called NXT (Fig. 2).

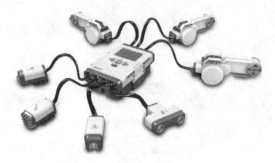

Fig. 2. NXT Microprocessor, sensors and mechanisms

The newly-built robots can, by using the correct programming tools, execute a set of actions and can react to stimuli received by their sensors. Lego Mindstorms are used as an educational tool to solve problems, being at the same time a pleasant and interesting occupation for the children. The children built their own constructions putting into practice their special skills, knowledge and abilities via a process of building, experimenting, giving feedback and trouble-shooting. Their distinct feature, which bears an added value, is that the students see them as more of a game, than as an educational tool, as the majority has already "played" with them since it is one of the first toys the children come in contact with since their early childhood (block constructions). The reasoning behind it is that the child should build the knowledge by themselves and that this is a very efficient educational process only when it comes directly through the game itself [5][6].

2.3   Methodology

The selection of the above tools is substantiated by the fact that they have been designed driven by the contemporary student-centered learning theories. App Inventor as well as Lego Mindstorms are based in the discipline of "constructivism" as developed by Jean Piaget [7] and as it was redefined by the philosophy of "constuctionism" by Seymour Papert[8][9]. The authors have developed the game according to the above theories setting the following objectives: a) forming the "new knowledge" to be more efficient through the children's involvement in constructing objects and/or entities that bear personal meaning, b)forming the correct learning environment which provides authentic activities engaging in solving open-problems in the real world, encouraging, therefore, the expression and personal involvement in the learning procedure, as well as supporting social interaction, and c) the problem to be solved should trigger the learning. In order for the children's interest to be sustained and for the atmosphere to be challenging children should incorporate their own experiences and desires in the class. So, the authors have developed the game presented in the following section based not only on the above methodology but also on the given appeal that the youths have towards smartphones and specifically towards mobile games.

3   Results and Discussion

In an attempt to put theory into practice a digital game has been designed and developed for android smartphones using the above technological tools always considering the contemporary learning theories. The application was entitled "NXTriviaRacing", screens of which are shown in Fig. 3.

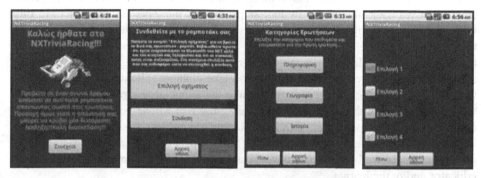

Fig. 3. NXTriviaRacing Application Screens

The title by itself states that it is a combination of quiz games (trivia) and racing along with the robotic constructions of Lego Mindstorms and NXT.

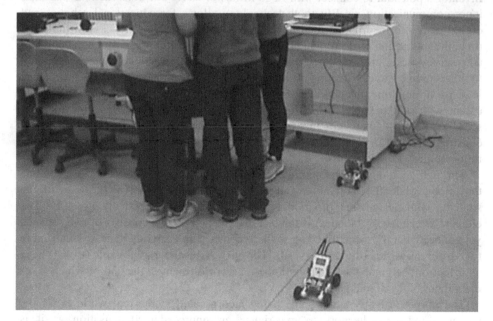

Fig. 4. Robotic vehicles in action. They were designed and constructed by the children.

According to the scenario, the player is called to answer knowledge trivia. In this case and bearing in mind the educational feature of the game, the questions are grouped in three categories (informatics, geography, history) with questions formed based on the curriculum of the according subjects of the Secondary School Grade A. The application is connected via Bluetooth with a robotic vehicle built by the students (Fig. 4).

Every correct answer sets the vehicle to motion in X steps, and every wrong answer moves back the vehicle by half steps, taking, thus, part in a car race. In this way, no Wrong or Right labels are used as the player understands by the motion if they answered right or wrong using the pedagogical theories of incentives and rewarding of the students. The questions are stored in a remote Database where the administrator has access so as to be able to make changes, alterations and additions. One can download them via a special button in the application screen. Every team has their own vehicle with the winning team being the one whose vehicle is ahead upon completion of the questions. "NXTriviaRacing" game is, first and foremost, an attempt to demonstrate the advantages of App Inventor as a programming environment, as well as its extensive possibilities for the ambitious programmer-educator and/or the learner.

An alternative realization would require more complicated commercial tools and specialized knowledge which are neither appealing nor fun for the majority of children or even adults who would be keen to create their own applications. App Inventor's potential to connect with Lego Mindstorms robotic constructions and their inner communication via Bluetooth technology allows for educational robotics and digital games to incorporate their advantages into the learning process. At the same time, the interaction of the digital game with robotic constructions, which the children themselves make, presents some distinctive characteristics and advantages compared to other mobile games. Creating a simple game for smartphones would not intrigue, at least for a long time, the children, since they have familiarized themselves to a great extent with similar games, which in many cases are highly appealing both for their scenario and for their graphics. However, if the game interacts with robotic constructions that the children themselves have made, then this is an entire different thing altogether.

Through a gaming procedure children go from players to co-creators of the game they play, while the motivation and the interest is multiplied in the case of the students who design and program it, something which is actually possible. The element which labels it distinct is the fact that the application consists of two separate yet connected at the same time games that interact with each other and are realized in two different worlds (digital-physical). The answers to the digital game (trivial) have an effect on the game taking place in the real world (racing), the end of which gives the winner of the digital game.

The purpose of the digital game being incorporated in the real world is for the students and the educators to experience an unprecedented sensation as it is completely different form the games they have been accustomed to so far and which will, on the one hand, intrigue their interest and curiosity and, on the other hand, will understand in practice that the programme can have an effect both on the digital and on the real world. To test the extent to which this is realizable in practice, in real classroom conditions, the opportunity was given to students of Grade A of Gravia Secondary School to play this game after they had built their own robotic vehicles. The results were more than satisfactory as there was great enthusiasm, eager participation, competition and determination to continue the game even through break time. Unfortunately and due to personalized information involving children's sensitive information, the respective video will not be available in social media channels.

The reactions spurred during the game indicated that the success of the game is mainly contingent to the fact that the children saw their answers to the game materialize into something totally different from what they had been used to. Even if they didn't win any points, they could still see the robotic vehicle that they had built themselves moving back and forth depending on their answers in a race where the winner is the one who would provide with the more correct answers. The success of this venture was more than evident in the agonizing faces of the children as they waited to see the "ramifications" of their answers.

4   Conclusions and Future Work

App Inventor and NXTriviaRacing were inspired by the indelible quest of the educator for ways to lead to the solution of the greatest "riddle" of all that today's educator is called upon to answer: provide the students with the correct "motivational tools" to actively participate in the learning process. App Inventor can give substantial answers, under specific circumstances, to their problem as it uses the most popular of all communicative devices amongst youths and other people, as well. Testing the game to students of Gravia Secondary School was a successful experiment and testifies that App Inventor's potential opens up new horizons as far as using games and robotics in the educational context. Notwithstanding, to get safest and conclusive results it is necessary to have field research using the above application anew, as such or modified by the students themselves during a school project and to further research the students thoughts and concerns via open-ended question polls.

Acknowledgements. "NXTriviaRacing" application as well as its trial at the mentioned school was part of a dissertation entitled "Incorporation and use of M.I.T. App Inventor in the educational process. NXTriviaRacing case-study" that took place within the Postgraduate Program entitled "Information and Communication Technologies for Education". The Program is supported by the Department of Early Childhood Education, the Department of Communication and Media (National and Kapodestrian University of Athens), the Department of Architecture (University of Thessaly), in partnership with the Department of Electronics of Technological Educational Institute of Piraeus.

References

1. Dewey, J.: Experience and Education. Touchstone Edition. Simon and Schuster, New York (1938, 1993, 1997) ISBN:0-684-83828-1
2. Prensky, M.: Digital natives, digital immigrants. On the Horizon 9(5) (2001a), http://www.marcprensky.com/writing/prensky%20-%20digital%20natives,%20digital%20immigrants%20-%20part1.pdf (last accessed: September 4, 2012)
3. Ofcom: Communications Market Report: UK (August 2011), http://stakeholders.ofcom.org.uk/binaries/research/cmr/cmr11/UK_CMR_2011_FINAL.pdf (last accessed: September 04, 2012)
4. Pew Research Center's Internet & American Life Project: Teens, Smartphones & Texting (2012), http://www.pewinternet.org/~/media//Files/Reports/2012/PIP_Teens_Smartphones_and_Texting.pdf (last accessed: September 04, 2012)
5. Hussain, S., Lindh, J., Shukur, G.: The effect of LEGO Training on Pupils' School Performance in Mathematics, Problem Solving Ability and Attitude: Swedish Data. Educational Technology & Society 9(3), 182–194 (2006), http://www.ebiblioteka.lt/resursai/Uzsienio%20leidiniai/IEEE/English/2006/ETSJ_2006_3_16.pdf (last accessed: October 15, 2012)
6. LEGO Dacta A/S. Study of Educational Impact of the LEGO Dacta Materials - INFOESCUELA – MED (1999), http://tinyurl.com/c7m87v6 (last accessed: November 28, 2012)
7. Piaget, J.: To Understand Is To Invent. Basic Books, N.Y. (1974), http://unesdoc.unesco.org/images/0000/000061/006133eo.pdf (last accessed: October 15, 2012)
8. Papert, S.: Mindstorms: Children, Computers, and Powerful Ideas. Basic Books Inc., New York (1980) ISBN:0-465-04627-4
9. Papert, S.: The Children's Machine. Basic Books Inc., New York (1993) ISBN:0-465-01830-0

Building Interactive Books Using EPUB and HTML5

Dimitris Gavrilis, Stavros Angelis, and Ioannis Tsoulos

Digital Curation Unit – IMIS, Athena Research Center, Artemidos 6 & Epidavrou,
Athens, Greece
{d.gavrilis,s.angelis}@dcu.gr, itsoulos@gmail.com

Abstract. The recent developments in the digital publishing domain have promoted the use of open formats for digital publishing. This paper presents a study that has been carried out using the EPUB 2.0 format along with HTML5 and JavaScript technologies showing how a digital book can embed HTML5 applications that interact with the user and report back to a publishing server (reader/student analytics).

Keywords: Digital publishing, epub, html5, analytics.

1 Introduction

The recent developments in the digital publishing domain have promoted the use of open formats for digital publishing. Now, books in the EPUB and PDF formats are read using internet tablets and smart phones and trends show they will replace traditional printed books much sooner than we think. The main reasons for this burst of electronic books, journals and newspapers are:

- The advances on mobile computing making mobile devices faster, more powerful and with better user experience
- The low cost of mobile devices
- The improved battery-life on mobile devices
- The lower cost of obtaining a newspaper / ebook in digital format
- The ability to transfer/copy a digital book to multiple media (smart phone, internet tablet, PC).
- The availability of tools (online translators, lexicons, annotations)

The major advantage of printed books and newspapers has always been the much better clarity when reading on paper. However, with the latest high-resolution screens found in high-end mobile devices this advantage is found in both sides.

1.1 The EPUB Format

The traditional EPUB 2.0 format consists of a set of xhtml files structured in folders and packaged using the zip format into a single file with an .epub extension. These folders contain the text (xhtml files), the styles (css file) and the multimedia files

C.T. Angelis, D. Fotiadis, and A.T. Tzallas (Eds.): AMBI-SYS 2013, LNICST 118, pp. 31–40, 2013.

(jpeg, png, mpeg etc) of the ebook. A file with an .opf extension is included, that contains descriptive information about the ebook and its contents in XML and a file with a .ncx extencion that contains the table of contents also in XML format. The protocol does not prohibit the inclusion of files like images, videos as long as they are defined in the OPF file. The OPF file contains the description of every part of the EPUB file.A simple example for this file is given below:

```xml
<?xml version="1.0"?>


<package version="2.0" xmlns="http://www.idpf.org/2007/opf" unique-
identifier="BookId">


<metadata xmlns:dc=http://purl.org/dc/elements/1.1/
xmlns:opf="http://www.idpf.org/2007/opf">
<dc:title>Pride and Prejudice</dc:title>
<dc:language>en</dc:language>
<dc:identifier id="BookId" opf:scheme="ISBN">123456789X</dc:identifier>
<dc:creator opf:file-as="Austen, Jane" opf:role="aut">Jane Austen</dc:creator>
</metadata>


<manifest>
<item id="chapter1" href="chapter1.xhtml" media-type="application/xhtml+xml"/>
<item id="stylesheet" href="style.css" media-type="text/css"/>
<item id="ch1-pic" href="ch1-pic.png" media-type="image/png"/>
<item id="myfont" href="css/myfont.otf" media-type="application/x-font-opentype"/>
<item id="ncx" href="toc.ncx" media-type="application/x-dtbncx+xml"/>
</manifest>


<spine toc="ncx">
<itemref idref="chapter1" />
</spine>


<guide>
<reference type="loi" title="List Of Illustrations" href="appendix.html#figures" />
</guide>


</package>
```

The NCX file contains the table of contents for the epub file and a relative simple example for this file is given below

```xml
<?xml version="1.0" encoding="UTF-8"?> <!DOCTYPE ncx PUBLIC "-//NISO//DTD ncx 2005-
1//EN" "http://www.daisy.org/z3986/2005/ncx-2005-1.dtd">


<ncx version="2005-1" xml:lang="en" xmlns="http://www.daisy.org/z3986/2005/ncx/">
<head> <!-- The following four metadata items are required for all NCX documents,
including those that conform to the relaxed constraints of OPS 2.0 -->
  <meta name="dtb:uid" content="123456789X"/> <!-- same as in .opf -->
  <meta name="dtb:depth" content="1"/> <!-- 1 or higher -->
  <meta name="dtb:totalPageCount" content="0"/> <!-- must be 0 -->
  <meta name="dtb:maxPageNumber" content="0"/> <!-- must be 0 -->
</head>


<docTitle>
  <text>Pride and Prejudice</text>
</docTitle>


<docAuthor>
  <text>Austen, Jane</text>
</docAuthor>


<navMap>
  <navPoint class="chapter" id="chapter1" playOrder="1">
    <navLabel>
      <text>Chapter 1</text>
    </navLabel>
    <content src="chapter1.xhtml"/>
  </navPoint>
</navMap>


</ncx>
```

2   Smart Digital Books

The term smart digital books refer to ebooks that can provide interactivity to their readers, gather data and report these data to a cloud based analytics engine. Examples of such applications could be found in the education sector where a geometry application could be embedded in the page of an ebook and can report back the student's results to the analytics server. The results could indicate the types of errors the student makes and suggest an alternative reading path (e.g. suggest another – more basic math ebook to read).

2.1   Overall Technical Architecture

In contrast with traditional approaches, the technical architecture of a smart digital publishing platform requires a central server component that the ebook can link to if/when needed along with a knowledge base that contains the details of the data exchange protocol the specific ebook will use.

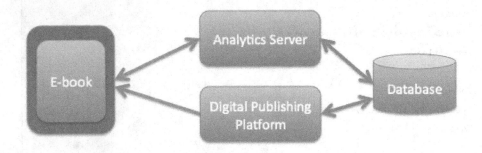

There are three main components found in the proposed architecture:

1. A database containing the ebooks, their metadata, a knowledge base of their sub-components (interactive tools)
2. A digital publishing platform containing all ebook information, information on members (e.g. students), book versions, etc. Through this server the client can buy/download the books, search the database, etc.
3. The analytics server is the primary component that receives information from the book itself. Information on opening the book, running one of the embedded applications and reporting back to the server if needed.

2.2   The Interactive Applications

An interactive application is a javascript/HTML5 based application which is embedded in the book on a single page. It is recommended that the application is embedded in a single page so that the re-flow component on the client does display the application on a single page. The application requires a set of libraries (javascript based) which should be defined under their own namespace/context and be included in the e-book thus can be run offline. A critical component in the application design is the one that handles communication with the analytics server. This particular component which we will focus on must take into account the following:

- Must be able to detect the presence of an Internet connection and consume all events if otherwise.
- Must be able to transmit all messages using the appropriate format for each application (JSON is the format used for information exchange).
- Must be able to periodically poll the analytics server for information (e.g. fetch relevant resources per page) but without interfering with the user's interaction with the ebook.

Each ebook transmits two types of messages (the type of message is encoded in the message header):
a) standard messages that transmit the page the user is on
b) messages that are application specific.

The message format is as follows:

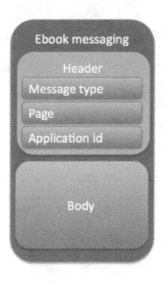

The message contains a message type (0=standard, 1=application).

The page contains the following array of values:
chapter, font-size, width, height, page number.
These values are used to determine the position in the ebook (pages vary due to different screen sizes, font-sizes etc.).

The application id

The body of the message which contains an array of key-value pairs which are application specific.

2.3   The Analytics Server

The analytics server handles all communication with the ebooks using a single data format (e.g. JSON). When the server receives a message, it queries the database for relevant resources and reports back with a reply message to the ebook. In the case of standard messages, usually relevant information is pulled from the database and is returned to the ebook. It is up to the ebook reader to display this information or not. In the event of an application sending a message, the analytics server decides whether to store that message and how to respond.

3   Implementation

The implementation of the above architecture has been carried out using PHP-MySQL on the server side (publishing platform and analytics server) and Java using android - sdk on the client (reader for android smart phones and tablets). The messaging system has been implemented using JSON protocol, which is widely used, simple yet powerful in terms of abstraction. As an example we present below a fraction only of the developed code needed to parse and display EPUB files in the android – sdk environment.

```
package EpubReader.com;
import android.app.Activity;
import android.os.Bundle
import java.io.IOException;
import java.io.InputStream;
import java.util.List;
import nl.siegmann.epublib.domain.Book;
import nl.siegmann.epublib.domain.Resource;
import nl.siegmann.epublib.domain.TOCReference;
import nl.siegmann.epublib.epub.EpubReader;
import android.app.Activity;
import android.content.res.AssetManager;
import android.graphics.Bitmap;
import android.graphics.BitmapFactory;
import android.os.Bundle;
import android.util.Log;
import android.view.Display;
import android.view.Gravity;
import android.view.View;
import android.webkit.WebView;
import android.widget.Button;
import android.widget.ImageButton;
import android.widget.ImageView;
import android.widget.TableLayout;
import android.widget.TableRow;
import android.view.View.OnClickListener;
public class EpubReaderActivity extends Activity {

        Bitmap coverImage=null;
        ImageView imgButton=null;
        Button homeButton=null;
        Button nextButton=null;
        Button prevButton=null;
```

```java
    ImageView img=null;
    WebView view=null;
     List<Resource> l;
     int currentPage=1;
@Override
public void onCreate(Bundle savedInstanceState) {
 super.onCreate(savedInstanceState);
 setContentView(R.layout.main);
 Display display = getWindowManager().getDefaultDisplay();
 int width = display.getWidth();
 int height = display.getHeight();
 AssetManager assetManager = getAssets();
 try {
  // find InputStream for book
  InputStream epubInputStream = assetManager
    .open("books/Dan.epub");
  // Load Book from inputStream
  Book book = (new EpubReader()).readEpub(epubInputStream);
  // Log the book's authors
  Log.i("epublib", "author(s): " + book.getMetadata().getAuthors());
  // Log the book's title
  Log.i("epublib", "title: " + book.getTitle());
  l=book.getContents();
  for(int i=0;i<l.size();i++)
  {
     Log.i("epublib","Data="+l.get(i).toString());
  }
  // Log the book's coverimage property
  coverImage = BitmapFactory.decodeStream(book.getCoverImage()
     .getInputStream());
  Log.i("epublib", "Coverimage is " + coverImage.getWidth() + " by "
     + coverImage.getHeight() + " pixels");
  // Log the tale of contents
  logTableOfContents(book.getTableOfContents().getTocReferences(), 0);
 } catch (IOException e) {
    Log.e(null, "adynamia anoigmatos arxeiou");
  Log.e("epublib", e.getMessage());
 }
 imgButton=(ImageView)findViewById(R.id.button1);
 imgButton.setImageBitmap(coverImage);
 imgButton.setClickable(true);

 homeButton=(Button)findViewById(R.id.button2);
 homeButton.setText("Home");
 homeButton.setOnClickListener(new OnClickListener()
```

```
{
    @Override
    public void onClick(View v) {
    currentPage=1;
    byte[] bytes = null;
                    try {
                            bytes=l.get(currentPage).getData();
                    } catch (IOException e) {
                            e.printStackTrace();
                    }
            String encoding=l.get(currentPage).getInputEncoding();
            String contentsHtml=new String(bytes);
            String type=l.get(currentPage).getMediaType().getName();
            view.loadData(contentsHtml, type, encoding);
            view.invalidate();
    }
});
prevButton=(Button)findViewById(R.id.button3);
prevButton.setText("Prev");
prevButton.setOnClickListener(new OnClickListener()
{
            @Override
            public void onClick(View v) {
            currentPage=currentPage-1;
            if(currentPage==0)
            {
                    currentPage=1;
                    return;
            }
             byte[] bytes = null;
             try {
                            bytes=l.get(currentPage).getData();
                    } catch (IOException e) {
                            e.printStackTrace();
                    }
            String encoding=l.get(currentPage).getInputEncoding();
            String contentsHtml=new String(bytes);
            String type=l.get(currentPage).getMediaType().getName();
            view.loadData(contentsHtml, type, encoding);
            view.invalidate();
    }
    });
nextButton=(Button)findViewById(R.id.button4);
nextButton.setText("next");
nextButton.setOnClickListener(new OnClickListener()
```

```
{

    @Override
    public void onClick(View v) {
            currentPage=currentPage+1;
            if(currentPage>=l.size())
            {
                    currentPage--;
                    return;
            }
             byte[] bytes = null;
              try {
                            bytes=l.get(currentPage).getData();
                      } catch (IOException e) {
                              // TODO Auto-generated catch block
                              e.printStackTrace();
                      }
         String encoding=l.get(currentPage).getInputEncoding();
         String contentsHtml=new String(bytes);
         String type=l.get(currentPage).getMediaType().getName();

                          view.loadData(contentsHtml, type, encoding);
                          view.invalidate();
                  }
});
view=(WebView)findViewById(R.id.webView1);
view.getSettings().setJavaScriptEnabled(true);
view.getSettings().setAppCacheEnabled(true);
view.getSettings().setJavaScriptCanOpenWindowsAutomatically(true);
byte[] bytes = null;
try {
            bytes=l.get(currentPage).getData();
        } catch (IOException e) {
                // TODO Auto-generated catch block
                e.printStackTrace();
        }
String contentsHtml=new String(bytes);
String encoding=l.get(currentPage).getInputEncoding();
String type=l.get(currentPage).getMediaType().getName();
view.loadData(contentsHtml, type,encoding);
view.loadUrl( "javascript:window.location.reload( true )" );  }

/**
 * Recursively Log the Table of Contents
 *
```

```
     * @param tocReferences
     * @param depth
     */
   private void logTableOfContents(List<TOCReference> tocReferences,
      int depth) {
   if (tocReferences == null) {
       Log.i("epublib","null toc");
     return;
   }
   Log.i("epublib","size of toc = "+tocReferences.size());
   for (TOCReference tocReference : tocReferences) {
     StringBuilder tocString = new StringBuilder();
     for (int i = 0; i <=depth; i++) {
       tocString.append("\t");
     }
     tocString.append(tocReference.getTitle());
     Log.i("epublib", tocString.toString());
     logTableOfContents(tocReference.getChildren(), depth + 1);
   }
 }
}
```

4   Conclusions

In this paper a smart ebooks architecture has been presented. This architecture has been designed based on the EPUB 2.0 protocol, it makes use of javascript and html5 technologies and a prototype application has been developed using Java on an android device (smart phone and tablet). On the server side, the server components have been implemented using open source tools: Php, MySQL, Apache. The preliminary results show the capabilities of real interactive ebooks and are very promising. Future work includes the use of a reasoning engine that will process the application messages.

References

1. http://en.wikipedia.org/wiki/EPUB
2. http://idpf.org/epub
3. Miller, B.N., Ranum, D.L.: Beyond PDF and ePub: toward an interactive textbook. In: ITiCSE 2012 Proceedings of the 17th ACM Annual Conference on Innovation and Technology in Computer Science Education, pp. 150–155 (2012)

Effects of Exercise in Diabetic Rats Using Continuous Wavelet Transform

Dimitrios G. Tsalikakis[1], Ioannis Nakos[2], Alexandros T. Tzallas[3], Evagelos Karvounis[4], and Markos Tsipouras[3]

[1] Research & Analysis Laboratory, Department of Informatics and Telecommunication Engineering, University of Western Macedonia, Kozani, Greece
[2] Biomedical Research Foundation, Academy of Athens, Center for Experimental Surgery, Athens, Greece
[3] Department of Informatics & Telecommunications Technology Technological Educational Institute of Epirus, Arta, Greece
[4] Department of Biomedical Research, Institute of Molecular Biology and Biotechnology-FORTH, Ioannina, Greece
dtsalikakis@uowm.gr, ioannisnakos78@gmail.com,
{atzallas,ekarvouni}@cc.uoi.gr, markos@cs.uoi.gr

Abstract. This paper explores an approach to study entropy differentiations of heart's activities estimation in Low Frequency (LF) and High Frequency (HF) bands. Dataset composed of 34 ECGs, obtained from healthy and diabetic rats under normal and exercise living conditions. RR intervals extracted efficiently in order to create Heart Rate (HR) time series. Continuous Wavelet Transform (CWT) has been used, as the most appropriate approach, to evaluate the effects of exercise on healthy and diabetic HR variability (HRV). Statistical analysis performed taking into account both wavelet entropy in the low and the high frequency selected bands and the corresponding index LF/HF of the wavelet coefficients. Our results show that wavelet entropy measure based on CWT decomposition can capture significant differences between the specific frequency regions that are intrinsically related to the structure of the RR signal. According to our analysis, diabetic rats living under exercise conditions appear to have a reduced LF/HF entropy ratio compared to healthy population.

Keywords: HRV, Diabetic, Exercise, Continuous Wavelet Transform, Wavelet Entropy.

1 Introduction

Over the last three decades, signal processing in biomedical field involve the analysis of measurements to extract useful information upon which physicians can make decisions. New ways of biomedical signal processing has been discovered using a variety of mathematical functions and algorithms. One very powerful tool that has been used for the analysis of such signal is the wavelet transform [1].

In normal conditions, there is a balance between the sympathetic and parasympathetic system known as the sympathovagal balance. The RR intervals, as

C.T. Angelis, D. Fotiadis, and A.T. Tzallas (Eds.): AMBI-SYS 2013, LNICST 118, pp. 41–49, 2013.
© Institute for Computer Sciences, Social Informatics and Telecommunications Engineering 2013

shown in Fig. 1, are the key of understanding the activity of the autonomic nervous system [2].

Changes in beat-to-beat heart rate calculated from Electrocardiograph (ECG), known as Heart Rate Variability (HRV) is under continuous research and it is being conducted with several new works. HRV allows the evaluation of the balance mentioned above and has been shown to be a predictor of the occurrence of cardiac dysfunctions [2].

Diabetes mellitus (DM) is a severe illness that has reached epidemic proportions worldwide. In particular, type II diabetes has increased significantly over the last years [3]. Patients with diabetes often develop cardiovascular diseases, like heart failure (HF) mainly caused from hypertension and coronary artery disease [4]. HRV decreases with diabetes and is associated with a high risk of cardiac arrhythmias, sudden death and an overall high mortality and morbidity rates. Exercise is an effective adjunct to pharmacological therapy of diabetes [5].

We decided to investigate this hypothesis by evaluating the entropy of HRV recordings. The estimation of entropy obtained from wavelets, providing a time-frequency representation of the signal with optimal time-frequency resolution. Wavelet entropy overcomes limitations as stationarity that fourier transform takes into account.

The application of wavelets in cardiology has been introduced with several approaches [6]. Detection of ischemia from QRS and identification of biological markers are some of the published applications [7]. All newest wavelet applications in ECG signals are reviewed lately in [8].

Especially, in time frequency analysis of HRV, different wavelet methods has been applied [9,10]. The idea of measure the wavelet entropy from CWT scales has used before in [11,12] and generally wavelets coefficients shown that could be a measure of power in frequency domain that suits to various medical applications [13].

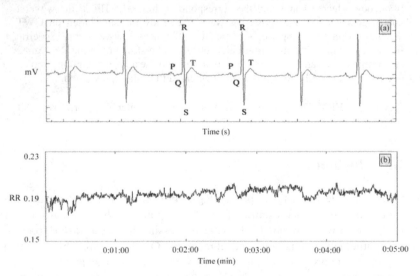

Fig. 1. This scheme demonstrates (a) An ECG graph from a healthy rat with the characteristic features and (b) RR series extracted from an ECG of a healthy rat

In this study, the CWT were utilized to extract and analyze wavelet entropy differentiations of HRV in high frequency (HF), very low frequency (VLF), ultra-low frequency (ULF) and low frequency (LF) bands. Objective of this paper was to evaluate the CWT based wavelet entropy to capture significant differences between the specific frequency regions. Another contribution of this work was to demonstrate the effects of exercise to the LF/HF energy healthy and diabetic subjects living under a daily workout program.

2   Methods

2.1   Wavelet

In the last few years, the wavelet transform has become an important tool in the field of HRV. Although the concept of the wavelets presented earlier, the first algorithm was developed in 1988 and since then many modification of wavelets has been published [14].

A wavelet is a "small wave" of small duration having an average value that is zero. Unlike fourier transform, where fourier sine and cosine functions are smooth, predictable and extend from minus to plus infinity, wavelets could be chosen from an unlimited tank of basis functions, they are usually non-symmetrical, with small duration and a finite period.

The decomposition of a signal using a wavelet transform needs a ψ function sufficiently regular and localized, called "Mother function". Wavelet transformation is a linear operation that decomposes the signal into a number of scales corresponding to frequency components and evaluates every scale with a certain resolution [15, 16].

The implementation of the WT results to a serial list of coefficients named wavelet coefficients, which represent the evolution of the correlation between the signal and the mother function at different levels of analysis (or different ranges of frequencies) all along the HRV series [17].

2.2   Continuous Wavelet Transform

Wavelet transforms categorized in essentially two distinct classes: the continuous wavelet transform CWT and the discrete wavelet transform DWT. Using a variable window width of mother function, related to the scale of observation, the CWT has the ability of isolation of the high frequency features. CWT advantage is to provide varying time-frequency resolution.

CWT that is applied to the signal s(t) defined as,

$$CWT(a,b) = \frac{1}{\sqrt{a}} \int_{-\infty}^{\infty} s(t)\psi\left(\frac{t-b}{a}\right) dt \tag{1}$$

Where $s(t)$ is the signal, $\psi(t)$ is the mother wavelet, a is the scaling parameter in y-axis, b is the shift parameter in x-axis and $1/\sqrt{a}$ is an energy normalization index which makes wavelets of dissimilar scale has the same amount of energy and t is the time. A wavelet family $\psi(a, b)$ is the set of elemental functions obtained from dilations and translations of a mother wavelet ψ.

There are several families of wavelet and each one has specific features. In our study, the choice of the basis function was Daubechies 6 (db6) and the selection made experimentally. The daubechies (db) wavelets have many advantages that make the db wavelets well suited for HRV analysis [18].

The RR signal was resampled at 10 Hz and the wavelet coefficients were calculated on sets of 5 minutes. If the signals included ectopic beats we removed them using a sliding window average filter. Then the sampled signals were interpolated using cubic spline interpolation and resampled in 4 Hz.

In CWT, frequency bands change with scales. We accept that the association of the center frequency F_c of the wavelet function, when the wavelet is dilated by a factor a, becomes F_c/a. Eventually, if the underlying sampling period of the signal is Δ, we also accept that the scale a is expressed as frequency from the equation 2.

$$F_a = \frac{F_c}{a\Delta} \tag{2}$$

The frequency F_a is inversely proportional to scale a. Large scale corresponds to a low frequency and small scales correspond to high frequencies providing details about the HRV signal.

Table 1. Frequency decomposition after CWT and the related scales

HRV Bands	Scales	Frequency (Hz)
ULF	36-124	0.101-0.02
VLF	14-35	0.27-0.102
LF	5-13	0.75-0.28
HF	1-4	3.65-0.90

Frequency decomposition and related scale range are listed in Table 1. After several trials we decided that using a 124 linear scales decomposition of CWT provides high resolution. The ULF band is localized in the scales 124-36, the VLF band in scales 35-14, LF band in 13-5 and the LF band in scales between 4-1.

2.3   Wavelet Entropy

The wavelet entropy (WE) has been proposed as a measurement to quantify the irregularity of a signal. In this study, we used it as a feature to study the effects of exercise conditions in healthy and diabetic rats.

To provide valuable information about these effects in the selected bands, we calculate the wavelet entropy using the wavelet coefficients $C_j(k)$ that correspond at each resolution level j.

For the calculation of energy at each time sample k we use the equation 3.

$$E(k) = \sum_{j=1}^{j} |C_j(k)|^2 \tag{3}$$

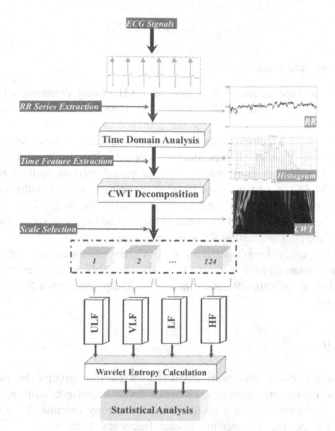

Fig. 2. The proposed method is presented for rat ECG signals. Generally, the first step involves the extraction of R peaks from the ECGs and the construction of RR series. At next step, time domain analysis provides several information for the signals such as beat-per-minute, mean values, standard deviation, etc. The CWT is then applied on the RR interpolated series and the wavelet entropy is computed at each scale. After calculation of the wavelet entropy at each corresponding frequency range the data is ready for statistical analysis.

While for the calculation of the total energy we consider the equation 4

$$E_{total} = \sum_{j=1}^{j} \sum_{k=1}^{N} |C_j(k)|^2 = \sum_j E_j \qquad (4)$$

Dividing the energy at a level j by its total energy is equivalent to define a probability distribution. So the energy in scales is defined from the equation 5, where the $\sum_j p_j = 1$ and the distribution p_j considered as time-scale density.

$$p_j = \frac{E_j}{E_{total}} \qquad (5)$$

At last, writing the well-known definition of wavelet entropy, wavelet entropy $H_{WT}(p)$ defined as in equation 6.

$$H_{WT}(p) = -\sum_{i=1}^{j} p_j \cdot log_2[p_j] \qquad (6)$$

2.4   Preprocessing Data

Telemetry ECGs were acquired at a rate of 1 kHz using commercially available hardware and software (Dataquest™ A.R.T. 4.0, Data Sciences International, Inc.). Baseline recordings were reviewed for the presence of arrhythmia and/or excessive movement artifacts and records containing such events were not analyzed further.

In this work, all the analysis procedure completed using custom algorithms which was developed in Matlab environment. The proposed method applied to a dataset composed of 34 ECGs, obtained by 24 hour recordings, form healthy and diabetic male Wistar rats under normal and exercise conditions. We select 5 min ECG segments from each group based on visual inspection of the most stable and rhythmic HR. After R wave peak extraction RR series generated.

As for the frequency-domain analysis of HRV, RR series were resampled by a 2nd order quadratic interpolation method at 10 Hz and NaN values removed. Power spectrum was obtained using Welch's method at 256 points with a 50% overlap and Hanning window.

3   Results

As we mentioned above, data were divided into the four groups (healthy, healthy under exercise conditions, diabetics, diabetics under exercise conditions) and CWT analysis was performed for each group. Wavelet entropy calculated for each group from the CWT scales that corresponds to each frequency domain.

In order to extract further information about from the data, classical time domain analysis and frequency analysis performed using custom algorithms as described in details previously [19]. We also calculate the RMS (Root Mean Square), the signal power contained in ultra-low, very low, low and high frequencies using the Welch method [19]. Using the RSM power, we calculate the index of LH/HF, which represents the sympathovagal balance of the heart.

Statistical analyses were performed to evaluate the ability of the wavelet energy to discriminate the effect of exercise in healthy and diabetic population of rats.

All data values normalized and the Analysis of Variance (ANOVA) was used to test the null hypothesis that there is no difference of the mean values of the index of LF/HF of the WE between the groups "healthy – healthy exercise" and "diabetes – diabetes exercise" by analyzing or comparing the sample variance of groups. Statistical significance was established at the $p<0.05$ level.

ANOVA test pointed out that between the groups healthy – healthy exercise and diabetes – diabetes exercise, low and high frequency components and the index HF/LF quantified by WE have significant differences. We also used ANOVA to test the hypothesis for the mean values of index LF/HF calculated from the RMS but the results show significant differences between the healthy and healthy exercise group but no significant differences between diabetic and diabetic exercise group.

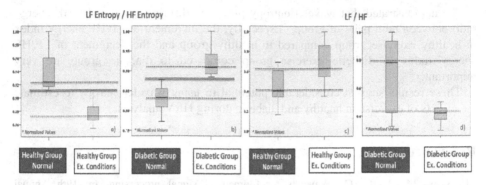

Fig. 3. Box-and-whisker plot of wavelet entropy (normalized) based on CW transform, computed for Healthy, Healthy under exercise, Diabetic and Diabetic under exercise conditions heartbeat intervals. The median for each group presented with the mark (−) in the box, the edges of the boxes are the 25th and 75th percentiles.

We present box-and-whisker plots of the index of LF/HF, calculated from the wavelet entropy from the CWT scales (Fig. 3(a), 3(b)) and from RMS (Fig. 3(c), 3(d)). In Fig. 3, box-and-whisker graphs show the distribution of the LF/HF using the lowest value, highest value, median value and the size of the first and third quartile. It is more clearly shown from the box-and-whisker plots in Fig. 3(a), 3(b) that exercise has notable effects the wavelet coefficients energy of the divided frequencies something that we didn't notice in power spectral indexes (LF and HF powers).

The results of this study showed that the index of LH/HF energy from wavelet coefficients significantly increased in normal subjects under exercise conditions compared with normal subjects. We also find out something very interesting. The index of LF/HF energy from CWT scales noticeable decreased in healthy rats under exercise conditions compared with healthy rats (Fig. 3(a), 3(b)). We couldn't get clearly the same results when we compare the LF/HF from RMS of the HRVs of the same groups as it can be shown in Fig. 3(c), 3(d).

The ANOVA method was also used to statistically test whether exercise conditions produced significant effects on the VLF and ULF bands derived from wavelet scales. Results demonstrated that there wasn't any significant difference in both pair of groups.

4   Conclusion

This study presents an approach based on CWT to estimate the impact of exercise in the wavelet entropy calculated from the wavelet coefficients in four frequency bands. ECGs collected from healthy and diabetic rats under normal and exercise conditions.

To discriminate the effect of exercise in healthy and diabetic population of rats statistical analyses were performed and the results presented with box-and-whisker plots.

We demonstrated that wavelet entropy produced discrimination in LF/HF energy ratio between both pairs of group. Especially, the increment of LF/HF energy index in healthy exercise group compared to healthy group and the decrement of LF/HF energy index in diabetic exercise group compared to diabetic group are very important.

These results suggest considerable potential in using wavelet entropy to estimate the effects of exercise in healthy and diabetic during HRV analysis.

References

1. Akay, M., Mello, C.: Wavelets for biomedical signal processing. In: 19th Annual International Conference of the IEEE Engineering in Medicine and Biology Society, vol. 6, pp. 2688–2691 (1997)
2. Stein, P.K., Kleiger, R.E.: Insights from the study of heart rate variability. Annual Review of Medicine 50, 249–261 (1999)
3. King, H., Aubert, R.E., Herman, W.H.: Global burden of diabetes, 1995–2025: prevalence, numerical estimates, and projections. Diabetes Care 21, 1414–1431 (1998)
4. Tuomilehto, J., Borch-Johnsen, K., Molarius, A., Forsen, T., Rastenyte, D., Sarti, C., Reunanen, A.: Incidence of cardiovascular disease in Type 1 (insulin-dependent) diabetic subjects with and with-out diabetic nephropathy in Finland. Diabetologia 41, 784–790 (1998)
5. Helmrich, S.P., Ragland, D.R., Leung, R.W., Paffenbarger, R.S.: Physical activity and reduced occurrence of non-Insulin-dependent diabetes Mellitus. New England Journal of Medicine 325, 147–152 (1991)
6. Couderc, J.P., Zareba, W.: Contributions of wavelets to non-invasive electro-cardiology. Ann. Noninvasive Electrocardiol. 3, 54–62 (1998)
7. Gramatikov, B., Thakor, N.: Wavelet analysis of coronary artery occlusion related changes in ECG. In: 15th Intern. Annual Conf. IEEE/EMBS, San Diego, p. 731 (1993)
8. Nagendra, H., Mukherjee, S., Vinod, K.: Application of wavelet techniques in ECG Signal processing: An overview. International Journal of Engineering Science and Technology 3, 7432–7443 (2011)
9. Jeong, Y.H., Su, K.L., Hong, B.P.: Denoising ECG using translation invariant multiwavelet. International Journal of Electrical and Electronics Engineering 3, 138–142 (2009)
10. Arvinti, B., Costache, M., Toader, D., Oltean, M., Isar, A.: ECG statistical denoising in the wavelet domain. In: 9th IEEE International Symposium of Electronics and Telecommunications, ISETC, Timisoara, pp. 307–310 (2010)
11. Quain, Q.R., Rosso, O.A., Basar, E., Schurmann, E.: Wavelet entropy in event-related potentials: a new method shows ordering of EEG oscillations. Biol. Cybern. 84, 291–299 (2001)
12. Bunluechokchai, S., English, M.J.: Detection of wavelet transform-processed ventricular late potentials and approximate entropy. IEEE Computers in Cardiology, 549–552 (2003)
13. Figliola, F., Serrano, E.: Analysis of physiological time series using wavelet transforms. IEEE Eng. Med. and Bio. Mag., 74–79 (1997)
14. Mallet, S.: A theory for multiresolution signal decomposition: the wavelet representation. IEEE Pattern Anal. and Machine Intell. 11 (1989)

15. Kadambe, S., Murray, R., Boudreaux-Bartels, G.F.: Wavelet transform - based QRS complex detector. IEEE Transactions on Biomedical Engineering 46, 838–848 (1999)
16. Li, C., Zheng, C., Tai, C.: Detection of ECG characteristic points using wavelet transforms. IEEE Transactions on Biomedical Engineering 42, 21–28 (1995)
17. Pichot, V., Roche, F., Gaspoz, J.M., Enjolras, F., Antoniadis, A., Minini, P., Costes, F., Busso, T., Lacour, J.R., Barthelemy, J.C.: Relation between heart rate variability and training load in middle-distance runners. Medicine and Science in Sports and Exercise 32, 1729–1736 (2000)
18. Daubechies, I.: The wavelet transform, time-frequency localization and signal analysis. IEEE Trans. Inform. Theory 36, 961–1005 (1990)
19. Oikonomidis, D.L., Tsalikakis, D.G., Baltogiannis, G.G., Tzallas, A.T., Xourgia, X., Agelaki, M.G., Megalou, A.J., Fotopoulos, A., Papalois, A., Kyriakides, Z.S., Kolettis, T.M.: Endothelin-B receptors and ventricular arrhythmogenesis in the rat model of acute myocardial infarction. Basic Research in Cardiology 2, 235–245 (2010)

Managing Children's Asthma with a Low Cost Web-Enabled Multifunctional Device

Ioannis Smanis[1], George Poursanidis[2], Pantelis Angelidis[1],
Alexandros T. Tzallas[3], and Dimitrios Tsalikakis[1]

[1] University of Western Macedonia,
Department of Informatics and Telecommunication Engineering, Greece
[2] University of Sussex, School of Engineering and Design
[3] Department of Informatics & Telecommunications Technology
Technological Educational Institute of Epirus, Arta
Greece
smanismech@icloud.com, poursang@gmail.com,
pantelis@media.mit.edu, atzallas@cc.uoi.gr, dtsalikakis@uowm.gr

Abstract. The essence of this paper is to present an innovative, viable, low cost, cloud based asthma management system solution, regarding children's asthma issues. The proposed device is a spirometric element that combines the functionality of several other devices that are so important for the daily life of asthma patients aged between 6 to 14. All the above are achieved using the latest technology in wireless and medical equipment that would make the device become irreplaceable to the end user.

Keywords: Asthma, Spirometer, Inhaler Detector, Wireless Module, Multifunctional.

1   Introduction

Asthma, is the most common reason patients visit pulmonologists in the US [1]. It is a chronic disease without permanent treatment. Patients with asthma have respiratory issues and they have to check their lungs status frequently. In a nutshell, it decreases the diameter of the lungs' airways and also produces a small amount of mucus that makes patients breath with difficulty. Dyspnea and coughing are the symptoms that follow patients through their entire life.

The daily medication for asthma consists of steroids in order to control the lungs' function [2]. This type of medication, includes the use of inhalers. The inhaler is a small form factor device that provides the user measured doses of the steroid which is placed into it. There is the blue colored inhaler, called reliever, for emergency asthma crisis and a red one called preventer, for daily use that improves and maintains the lungs' airways in good condition.

Moreover, there are some other devices that experts recommend for daily use. The spacer, peak flow meter and the spirometer:

C.T. Angelis, D. Fotiadis, and A.T. Tzallas (Eds.): AMBI-SYS 2013, LNICST 118, pp. 50–64, 2013.
© Institute for Computer Sciences, Social Informatics and Telecommunications Engineering 2013

The Spacer is a device that works in conjunction with the inhaler in order to help patients breathe the steroids in low pressure. It helps people to breathe easier than using the inhaler directly into their mouth.

The Peak Flow Meter measures the maximum level of a forced expiratory. It is quite useful for doctors due to the fact that it indicates in which colored health zone the patient belongs to [3]. There are three zones: the green zone is the healthier zone that patient do his usual activities without problems, the yellow zone describes some small breathing issues and patient cannot complete all of his daily activities and the red zone for emergencies in which patients cannot breath very well and need to move to a hospital. Contrary to spirometers that doctors use to monitor lungs' condition, peak flow meter is a cheap spirometer that measures only the peak of the expiratory air flow rate parameter (PEF) but it's still useful.

The Spirometer is the most advanced method of monitoring lungs function. Experts use many kinds of spirometers depending on the situation. The most prevalent type of spirometer is the digital spirometer. It's an electronic spirometer without mechanical parts that measures several medical parameters such as PEF (Peak Expiratory Flow), FVC (Forced Vital Capacity), FEFx (Forced Expiratory Flow rate in x percentage), FEV (Forced Expiratory Volume in t timeslot), FIFx (Forced Inspiratory Flow in x percentage). It has a built-in LCD screen and a wireless communication technology so that you can see and transmit the values of those parameters. They are required by doctors' diagnosis and they help them to make sure about patients health.

Currently, the devices mentioned above, are quite complex and expensive, hence they are unattractive to the end user. The cost of modern commercial spirometers can be over nine hundred dollars. They have screens, buttons, weird design and ugly interfaces that patients are at least reluctant to use, and quite user unfriendly, so they need to read many manual pages in order to operate them correctly.

In this paper, we describe a new way to address this problem, developing a novel spirometric device that could look more elegant and ergonomic. The external design must be attractive in order to use it more frequently during the day. Asthma is a disease that can easily affect younger people than 15 years old because of the vulnerable immunogenic system. Henceforth, they need more daily health monitoring than older people. Also, the prevalence and severity of childhood asthma have increased substantially in recent years [5]. This is the reason why the proposed device is focused to be used by children between 6 and 14 years old. Nowadays, children's daily life includes many activities that require a lot of energy. The biggest concern about children from 6 to 14 years old is finding a way to motivate children to use all the above-mentioned equipment every time and how difficult is to carry around them complex devices. It is quite obvious that we should motivate young children with asthma to use all these devices more frequently than they do presently.

2   Motivation

The main objective of this study is to develop a telemedicine system which can manage asthma data for patients in childhood without the need of frequent visits at health care centers. This system includes the development of a multi-functional spirometric device that can solve the problem of daily patient's monitoring. This study is about developing a novel device that could replace all current medication and monitoring devices with one single device being an essential part of a remote medical monitoring service. This device should combine a spirometer with peak flow meter and spacer because we should motivate children to be more responsible with their medication, while having fun playing with it at the same time.

A key feature that could motivate and train children about asthma and their lungs' function is the cooperation of the spirometer with devices as a smartphone or a tablet giving opportunities to mobile software developers to build game applications in order to motivate children to learn more about their health status. Finally, this device must be a relatively low cost product in order to succeed in our task. It is quite important, to make as affordable as we can, so it can be useful and attractive for parents who have children with asthma.

3   The Proposed Model

Using the proposed system, we can easily monitor patients through the Internet as a cloud based service. This system comprises of two devices and an internet service (Fig.1). The basic device is the spirometer that collects patient's measurements and data. The second device is a smart handheld device that plays a dual role in our model.

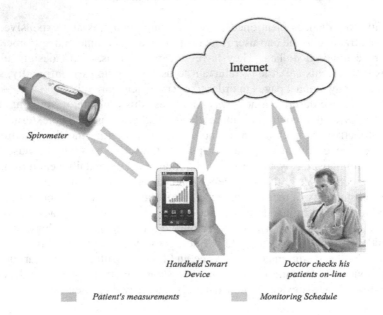

Fig. 1. This model can be the structure of an asthma telemedicine system with a cloud telemedicine service

The basic reason that we use a smart handheld is that spirometer can gain access to the internet through it via a Bluetooth wireless connection. Furthermore, an application is installed on the handheld with a simple to use interface. It contributes to manage the saved data in spirometer's memory and send them to doctor's monitoring system via a cellular or Wi-Fi connection. The app has the ability to display the current measurements and draw a real-time air flow graph when the child blows across the spirometer.

The Concept Works in a Quite Simple Manner

The child uses the spirometer during the whole day according to a predefined monitoring schedule.

When the device finds any previous paired smart device bluetooth enabled, it automatically establishes a connection. Then it launches a specific app showing the daily results and uploads them to a specific server which can only be accessed by the doctor. After that, patient's medical file is updated with new measurements.

Consecutively, the doctor can study his patient's health improvement and suggest a new monitoring schedule for the next days. So, he can upload a new schedule data to the spirometer via his information system. A sound alert will notify user that he must do a spirometric measurement or time to breathe the preventer steroid. Consequently, it's an interactive model, in which there is an interactive communication between spirometer and doctor.

We focus on developing a multi-functional spirometer as part of that telemedicine system with some concrete and discrete characteristics:

- *Elegant and simple design*
- *Reliable measurement ability*
- *Wireless connectivity with smart devices and computers*
- *Rechargeable*
- *Small and comfortable size and weight*
- *Easy to use UI (user experience)*
- *Visual and audio indications*
- *Invisible function to the user*
- *low cost (up to 250$)*

All these characteristics are our goals and guidelines in designing a useful medical device for monitoring asthma patients. We should implement an efficient architecture and set out specific technical features to reach the initial goals.

Starting to explain the functionality of the spirometer, we have to describe the basic architecture.

4 Architecture

The architecture of this spirometer should include some very remarkable features in order to achieve our requirements:

Features:

1. **Reliable Airflow sensor**
2. **LED indication** *for current airflow levels*
3. **Sound alerts**
4. **Inhaler detection**
5. **GPS** *for acquiring location data and geolocation*
6. **RTC** *for acquiring the time of an event*
7. **EEPROM Memory bank** *for saving monitoring schedule and measurement event data.*

Our project's target group is ages between 6 to 14 years old and it's impossible to carry around with them devices as a smartphone. Thus, we don't use the already smart devices' embedded stuff; we have to implement geolocation features, real time clock and a memory module into the device for better monitoring. The basic implementation architecture is illustrated in Fig. 2.

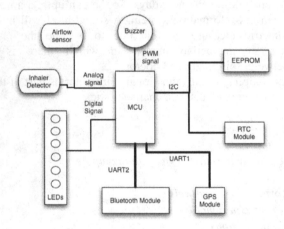

Fig. 2. This scheme constitutes the whole architecture which shows how all the basic electronic components communicate with central microcontroller

EEPROM memory and Real-Time-Circuit are connected with a microcontroller by an I2C synchronous serial interface. The Bluetooth and GPS module communicates through asynchronous UART protocol. An airflow sensor and a color sensor (thus the inhaler detector) are attached to analog inputs of the microprocessor in order to have better control at sampling procedure. The LED array and the buzzer are used as optical indication and sound notification respectively. They constitute the unique mechanism that children get feedback from the device in a simple way.

When the device is on, the microcontroller can be triggered by two ways. The one way is that users' blows, an air flow sensor detects elemental amount of air stream, then air flow samples are being saved in the memory IC as well as the time and date data. Then, the microcontroller asks for location determination from the GPS module and saves its data at the same memory IC. The second scenario is about the detection of a mounted inhaler. When the color sensor detects the existence of a blue or red color, microcontroller asks for location and time information again. The detection of each colored inhaler can be done as the plugged inhaler on the front of the spirometer reflects a unique color direct to the sensor's sensitive point. Then, the microcontroller saves a specific color value for each inhaler to the created event file.

Spirotube
Beyond the implementation part of the electronics, we need to design carefully an airway that airflow sensor will take the pressure samples when someone blows into the device. This procedure is very essential as the spirotube is the main hardware part that delivers two different samples of the inserted air flow to the airflow sensor. We can estimate the velocity of the air in liters/second via the output voltage of the airflow sensor and the following equation:

$$F_A = F_{FS} \left(\frac{V_O}{V_S} - 0.5 \right), \tag{1}$$

F_A = Flow applied across the device, F_{FS} = Full scale flow specified for the device,

V_O = Output voltage of the device, V_S = Supply voltage measured at the device.

Moreover, the spirotube is the contact between the user's mouth and the airflow sensor (Fig.3). It is designed with precision so as to achieve 150 Pa/L/sec airway resistance per 14 litters per second air velocity. That is the requirement of the ATS(American Thoracic Society) in standardization of spirometry.

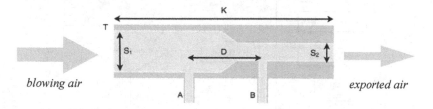

Fig. 3. Splinted view of the spirotube. In designing stage, we decided to make an asymmetric structure of the tube, building two different holes so as to increase the pressure drop across the fitting A and B. As we can see the S_1 diameter is bigger than the S_2 so as the pressure at the point A is enough increased than at the point B.

After real airflow tests [2], we have estimated that the suitable drop is 3/8" from the large S_1 diameter to the smaller S_2. This diameter drop is so crucial that the airflow sensor can clearly distinguish the pressure difference across the fittings without ambient interference.

Block Diagram

We should describe the full functionality of the ideal spirometer in the following block diagram (Fig. 4):

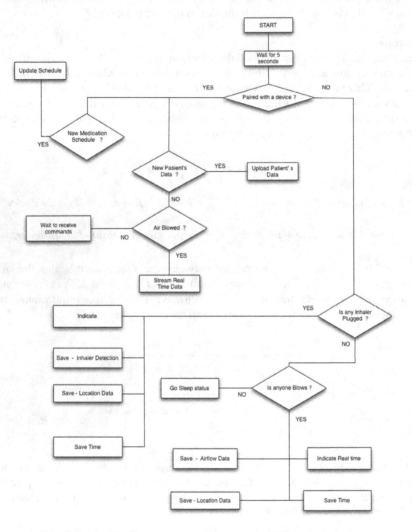

Fig. 4. Logic data flow diagram of the proposed spirometric device

When the spirometer is turned on, there an interval waiting time that device loads its program and the Bluetooth module searches for previously paired Bluetooth devices to establish a wireless connection. Actually, the first time that you will try to set up the spirometer, you need to engage a pairing process which takes no more than 5 seconds. In case of a successful connection with a smartphone for example, the spirometer can be updated with new medication or monitoring schedule by a specific application. If it's in use without wireless connection, data as a detected inhaler or air flowed, location and time would be saved in the built-in memory. All these data will be synced with doctor's files by a smart device internet connection.

5   Developing a Prototype

The chameleon prototype constitutes a simple combination of the basic materials and electronics building a simple digital spirometer. It includes only the most significant parts: airflow sensor, inhaler detector, LED indications, sound buzzer, bluetooth module and the power supplying circuits. A spirotube is built into the plastic enclosure (Fig.5).

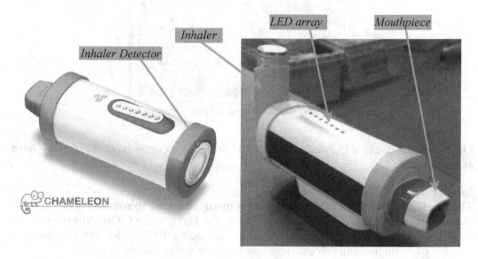

Fig. 5. Chameleon, the first extremely low cost spirometer prototype. In the left picture is showed the 3D rendered model and the one at right photo is pictured the real 3D printed construction. It's made by Asthma Management team with a cost of about 120$ during a two weeks innovation event in MIT Media Lab. *(27/01/2012)*

AirFlow Sensor
As an airflow sensor we have selected a differential pressure sensor that contains two different MEMS(MicroElectoMechanical Systems) based pressure sensor made by Honeywell. It operates comparing to different air samples and an internal circuit estimates the pressure difference between them and it exports an analog signal. There are three pins: the first is the analog voltage output and the other two of them for supplying purposes. We selected Honeywell Zephyr series the 3.3 Volt analog version in order to control the sampling rate via a central microcontroller.

It's the most expensive part of our implementation because of its high accuracy reaching at ±2.5%. It fits the ATS spirometry requirements being capable ranging air flow between 0 to 14 litters per second. Also, there is no need for calibration procedure and its low power consumption allows portable application use such as a spirometer. Concluding, there is no need to have any special requirements regarding extreme heat - which can be found in several African countries.

Breathing Tests Applied and Monitored

This Honeywell sensor is already pre-calibrated by the manufacturer. However we confirmed its operating condition via our digital oscillator performing some real-time blowing tests (Fig.6).

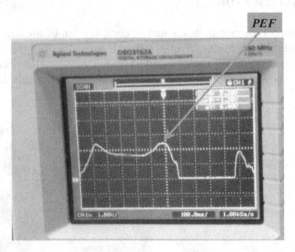

Fig. 6. Easily recognized PEF factor reaches 3.35 volts, the upper bound of the output voltage as we expected

Inhaler Sensor

The essential information when an inhaler is mounted on the spirometer is the color of the inhaler. So, we need a RGB color sensor as the Hamamatsu C9303 like the one we have used in our prototype. The C9303 is an analog RGB color sensor which is capable of distinguishing color differences between a vast variety of colors.

Moreover, it is suitable for our prototype because of its operating voltage ranging between 2.7 and 5.5 volts. The only issue is that it requires 3 ADC channels from the main chip, one for each basic color. Its small dimensions provide us with more flexibility to eliminate the wasted internal space by the electronic components.

The 3 output pins drive to the ADC chip the corresponded values of voltage for each color assisted by the light of a small white LED bulb. Then, the main chip calculates which color has the inhaler combining the three different values of the output voltage.

Main Chip

The main microcontroller was the PIC16F877A that operates as an Analog-to-Digital converter for 10 bit per sample with 625KHz sampling frequency. We supply this IC via a 5 volts circuit and a crystal oscillator at 20MHz. It constitutes a low power consumption MCU (MicroController Unit) that could be powered by a 2 volts source at least. It consumes less than 0.6 mA at 4MHz and 3 Volts Vcc (Fig. 7).

It is configured to release 4 analog input channels, 3 for the color sensor and one for the airflow sensor. A serial UART channel set up at 115.2kbps speed so as to communicate with bluetooth wireless module. That Microchip MCU applies the central management of the whole product. It sensors data based on the block diagram's flow. MCU is the only component that determines when the data should be saved or sent to wireless module.

Moreover, the main chipset blinks the LED array indicating notification about new monitoring schedule or corresponding to percentage level of the current expirations into the spirotube. The sound buzzer is driven by PWM pulses that are generated by an internal comparator varying frequency and duty cycle.

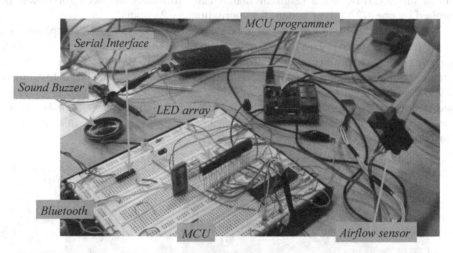

Fig. 7. All the electronic components pined on the breadboard . Testing the functionality of the whole circuit being the base of our final prototype.

Bluetooth Module

The first prototype was implemented via a CSR BC417 Bluetooth 2.1 EDR module. The converted air flow samples are delivered from the MCU to the module by a UART channel. After that, the data are transmitted wirelessly at 2.4GHz. Its power requirements are quite low. It operates at 3.3 volts and consumes 50mA at the maximum wireless transmit rate (2Mbps). Initially, we have set up for the HID Bluetooth profile for testing purposes and we achieved to send sensor's data to a terminal client computer application as it is revealed from the Fig. 8.

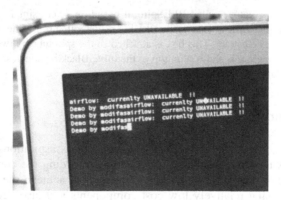

Fig. 8. Data wirelessly transmitted to terminal client of our computer by the first chameleon prototype via when it was turned on and paired

The second prototype is called BLESpiro. It is essentially a stripped down simple spirometer using Bluetooth 4.0 implemented via BLE profile. That is a significant improvement of the chameleon prototype decreasing the power consumption. It is the latest technology module that contributes in personal area networking and consumes current under 27mA. As a result of that it can eliminates the need for power be supplied by one 1/2AA type battery for approximately 24 hours.

The Bluegiga BLE112 bluetooth module is the most essential component on which the BLESpiro is based (Fig 9). The BLE112 module manages to replace multiple components as the microcontroller unit, ADC unit, supplying circuits and the wireless communication module in one single device. It utilizes the Texas Instrument CC2540 as integrated MCU chipset. Embedded 32 MHz and 32.678 kHz crystals are used for clock generation. The internal ADC is configured to 500KHz using resolution of 12bit per sample. BLE112 can approach the speed of 1Mbps for transmitting data over the air.

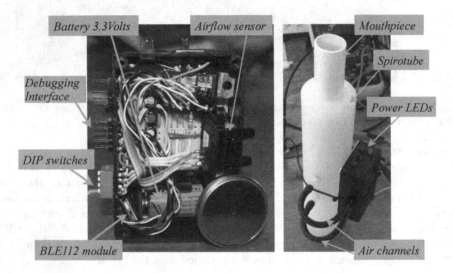

Fig. 9. The second prototype called BLESpiro, it based on a very simple structure. The small black box contains the airflow sensor, the BLE112 Bluetooth 4.0 module, our debugging PCB and a 1/2AA type 3.3V battery. This box is attached to the spirotube by two micro tubes 3mm. Also, a carton mouthpiece is showed on top of the tube. Black box enclosure is compared with a 3V coin cell battery.

6   Cost and Efficiency Ratio

A very important aspect of every new project that has aspirations in becoming the new standard is to make a quantitative research regarding the cost of the proposed system. It is quite obvious that we have managed to achieve the best performance possible, while using relatively low cost components and also keeping in mind the reliability of the system (Table I).

Table 1. The cost list of the real components that could be used for this project is shown below

Component description	Cost ($ USD)
Microcontroller (Microchip)	2-3
Airflow sensor (Honeywell)	70 - 90
Color sensor (Hamamatsu)	5
Bluetooth module (CSR)	8
Rechargeable Battery 3.7V	14-17
USB charging circuit	10
Electronic components	6-8
Spirotube made by Nylon/PVC	10-20
3D printed model	20-25
GPS module	26-27
EEPROM memory (Microchip)	1.5-3
RTC module	3.7-4
LEDs (9 pieces)	0.10
Piezo-electric Buzzer	1
PCB manufacturing	5-7
Total Cost	182.3 - 228.1

It is evident from the BOM's total cost, that the proposed device while keeping the price at a very low point, manages to implement more asthma devices in a single spirometric tool and all that at 230$. As a comparison, modern spirometers that are targeted to clinicians and experts are priced at around 1000$ and have only a fraction of our device's functionality.

Ultimately, the mass production of our device will reduce the total cost even further, hence the cost efficiency ratio will be even larger. The key part of our project, which is the Honeywell airflow sensor will be a lot cheaper in large quantities. Although it is one of the most expensive in its category, it manages to outperform the competitors by quite a margin and also enable us to use cheaper components for the other functions, thus, keeping the cost at a bare minimum.

7   Conclusion

The main objective of this project is to build from the ground up a multifunctional spirometric device for children aged between 6 to 14, with a cost concern and an interest to spearhead above the current offers even from reputable and well established manufacturers.

Thus, in this study, we are presenting a really low cost spirometer, extremely useful and with a user interface that would attract young children aged 6 to 14 which was our main goal for this project. Not only we managed to do that, but we also chose and implemented materials that are relatively cheap but tested, robust and quite reliable, which is also another goal that we have set from the beginning. It would be without cause if we managed to use cheap materials in our BOM, but made the device unreliable, which would end up being another toy for the child. This is not the case though. The ease of use of the device is evident and also it being small and user friendly, so that it will motivate the users to continuously challenge themselves.

There are several matters that should be taken into perspective though. The project was more or less self-funded although the final results were remarkable. It attracted the first price of the MIT Health and Wellness Innovation 2012 award, and got the applaud of many academics and companies related to the medical instrument industry.

We managed to pull through a wide variety of issues and provided a reliable, cheap, easy to use, all around replacement tool for most of the asthma issues that a patient faces every day in his life.

References:

1. http://www.nhlbi.nih.gov/health/health-topics/topics/asthma/treatment.html (last accessed October 13, 2012)
2. http://www.patient.co.uk/health/inhalers-for-asthma (last accessed November 21, 2012)
3. http://www.mayoclinic.com/health/asthma/DS00021/DSECTION=tests-and-diagnosis (last accessed November 05, 2012)
4. http://emedicine.medscape.com/article/137501-overview   (last accessed November 19, 2012)
5. Osborne, S.: Airways Resistance and Airflow through the Tracheobronchial Tree
6. Glynn, J., Schaefer, J., Bremer, A., Dias, A.: Low-Cost Spirometer, May 8 (2009)
7. Third National Health and Nutrition Examination Survey III, Spirometry Procedure Manual,Westat Inc.,1650 Research Boulevard Rockville, MD 20850 (301) 251-1500 (August 1988)
8. Lim, J.P.-K., Warwick, W.J., Hamen, L.G.: Pulmonary Function Measurement Using Flow Time Monitor (1998)
9. van Schalkwyk, E.M., Schultz, C., Joubert, J.R., White, N.W.: Guideline for Office Spirometry in Adults, 2004. South African Thoracic Society Standards of Spirometry Committee (2004)
10. Lin, C.-W., Wang, D.-H., Wang, H.-C., Wu, H.-D.: Prototype Development of Digital Spirometer (1998)
11. American Thoracic Society, Medical Section of the American Lung Association, Standardization of Spirometry, 1994 Update, This Official Statement of the American Thoracic Soclm WAS Adopted by the ATS' Board of Directors, November 11 (1994)
12. Agarwal, V., Ramachandran, N.C.S.: Design and development of a low-cost spirometer with an embedded web server (2008)
13. Fishman, A.P.: Pulmonary Diseases and Disorders, 2nd edn., vol. 3. McGraw-Hill Book Co., New York (1998)
14. Schiller, J.S., Lucas, J.W., Ward, B.W., Peregoy, J.A.: Summary Health Statistics for U.S. Adults: National Health Interview Survey (2010)

Appendix

Sample of the MCU Program Code

(Programming language Embedded C - MicroC compiler)

```c
void main() {
    ADCON0 = 0b10000101; // configuration MCU - ADC - CLOCK
    ADCON1 = 0b10001000; // configuration MCU - PORTS
    TRISA = 0xFF; // configuration port directions
    TRISB =0; // configuration port directions
    TRISC = 0b10000000; // configuration port directions
    UART1_Init(115200); //Initialize UART module at 115200bps
    Delay_ms(100); // Wait for UART module to stabilize
    Sound_Init(&PORTC, 3); // set up the buzzer port
    while (1) {
rawdata = ADC_Read(0); //Get 10-bit results of AD conversion
voltage=(((rawdata)/1023.0)*5*1000); //Voltage is in mV
airflow=400*((voltage/3300)-0.5)/0.4 //conversion formula(1)
percentage = (voltage-2000)/5; // percentage flow value
                                // for LEDs array use
digit = percentage % 10u;
digit1 = mask1(digit);
digit = (char)(percentage / 10u) % 10u;
digit10 = mask1(digit);


// capture value for each color via the color sensor
voltageR=(((ADC_Read(1))/1023.0)*5*1000);
voltageG=(((ADC_Read(2))/1023.0)*5*1000);
voltageB=(((ADC_Read(3))/1023.0)*5*1000);
```

```
// check which inhaler is mounted and send data
if (voltageR=<1020) and (voltageG=<1020) and
(voltageB=>1500 and voltageB=<3345)) {
Inhaler=Blue;
PORTB.RB2=0;
PORTB.RB3=1;
UART1_Write(Inhaler);
}
else if (voltageR=<1020) and (voltageG=<1020) and
(voltageB=>1500 and voltageB=<3345)) {
Inhaler=Red;
PORTB.RB2=1;
PORTB.RB3=0;
UART1_Write(Inhaler); }
else { Inhaler=None; UART1_Write(Inhaler); }
GO_DONE_bit = 0 ;
UART1_Write(10);
UART1_Write(13);
UART1_Write_Text("you blow");
UART1_Write(airflow); // send airflow sensor data via
//UART-bluetooth module
UART1_Write_Text("SCCM");
PORTB=0b10000000;
}
```

Integration of eHealth Service
in IPv6 Vehicular Networks

Sofiane Imadali[1], Athanasia Karanasiou[2], Alexandru Petrescu[1], Ioannis Sifniadis[2],
Eleftheria Vellidou[2], and Pantelis Angelidis[3]

[1] CEA, LIST, Communicating Systems Laboratory, 91191 Gif-sur-Yvette CEDEX, France
{sofiane.imadali,alexandru.petrescu}@cea.fr
[2] Vidavo Technical Department, Vidavo S.A., Thermi, Thessaloniki 57001, Greece
{it,helpdesk,projects}@vidavo.gr
[3] Wireless Sensors Laboratory, University of Western Macedonia,
Karamanli & Lygeris, Str Kozani 50100, Greece
pantelis@vidavo.gr

Abstract. Several convenience and efficiency applications have been proposed as part of recent vehicular networks (a.k.a. VANET) activities. Among these proposals, eHealth has often been studied as a time-critical application to emulate an ambulance. The Vehicle-To-Infrastructure (V2I) setting is the typical communication scenario to carry out the data in this case. From a user perspective, combining vehicular networking and eHealth to record and transmit a patient's vital signs is a special telemedicine application that helps hospital resident professionals to optimally prepare the patient's admittance. The current proposal pro-vides an IPv6 vehicular platform which integrates eHealth devices and allows sending captured user health-related data to a Personal Health Record (PHR) application server on the IPv6 Internet. The collected data are viewed remotely by a doctor and supports diagnostic decision. The resulting platform is then compared to the state-of-the-art related architectures.

Keywords: Vehicular networks, eHealth, IPv6, Testbed Integration, Remote diagnosis.

1   Introduction

Intelligent Transportation Systems (ITSs) [5] are envisioned to play a significant role in the future, making transportation safer and more efficient. As it was concisely stated at the Intelligent Transportation System World Congress in 2008: save time, save lives [1]. In order to achieve these objectives, V2I interactions have evolved to include various applications, some of which are safety-related and others user-oriented (infotainment).

1.1   M2M Devices Proliferation

According to some estimates, the size of the Internet doubles every 5.32 years, which will lead to an average of 6.58 connected devices per person by 2020 [6]. These 50

C.T. Angelis, D. Fotiadis, and A.T. Tzallas (Eds.): AMBI-SYS 2013, LNICST 118, pp. 65–80, 2013.
© Institute for Computer Sciences, Social Informatics and Telecommunications Engineering 2013

billion things [7] connect to the network in order to gather and spread information for various and unattended applications supporting new markets [8]. From an addressing perspective, these new and exciting opportunities come with the requirement of a larger addressing space. The current IPv4 addressing pool is nearly exhausted [9], which urges the transition to the new version of Internet Protocol (IPv6) giving the important numbering space it comes with (2^{96} times bigger than IPv4's) [10].

In the wide field of health informatics, eHealth is about the use of Internet to disseminate health related information [11]. The World Health Organization (WHO) defines eHealth as "the transfer of health resources and healthcare by electronic means". This activity includes the delivery of health information to health professionals and health consumers through the Internet and telecommunications in order to improve public health services. To be accurate, another term, mHealth, is defined as the subset of eHealth that concerns health services by means of mobile technologies such as mobile phones and PDAs (personal digital assistants) [2]. Health-related information is captured by small and various M2M devices and stored in large databases to be further processed in order to support diagnostics. The final goal is to improve efficiency and save lives [12].

1.2   IPv6 Vehicular Networking

Several years of research initiatives in the field of automotive applications proved the considerable improvement of traffic safety and new unattended market opportunities these applications could provide. eHealth is only one application example that could apply to the vehicular paradigm. V2I and V2V environments include several other examples of safety and service or infotainment applications support. Basically, we can classify these applications in two major categories: safety-oriented or user-oriented [13]. Safety applications are clearly time-critical tasks, where message delivery with short delay guarantee is the first design goal. To satisfy the time stringent requirement, non-IP (radio) communication technologies are often preferred over best-effort networks (Internet) for their reliability and reduced overhead[14]. Radio communications are initiated on dedicated channels [1]. In contrast, user-oriented applications are non-time-critical tasks, in which falls infotainment and other prevention on road applications. The use of Internet Protocol (best effort) to extend the supported geographic area for these applications is possible [15].

As we experience an upgrade in the Internet Protocol from version 4 to 6, the use of IPv6 in current standardization work for vehicular communications technologies guarantees a better integration in the Future Internet and ensures a better compatibility with unattended applications. For example, UMTS and LTE technologies support IPv6 according to 3GPP specifications [16], which opens new V2I services perspective using the deployed infrastructure, and this before the wide adoption and deployment of dedicated Roadside Units (RSUs) [17]. In recent ETSI activities, a GeoNetworking protocol combined with IPv6 has been experimented and standardized [15]. In the GeoNet project, a safety oriented application using broadcast has been defined. GeoBroadcasting is the use of relay messages from vehicle to vehicle (V2V) in a certain geographic neighborhood (zone or area) over IEEE 802.11p radio technology.

1.3   Heterogeneous Technologies

Wireless communication technologies such as ZigBee, Bluetooth, and WiFi are already widely used in the M2M industry and expected to be widely deployed in near future automotive communications. Limited computing and networking capabilities devices (including eHealth devices) are expected to use such means of communication with the outside world. These short range communication technologies are much more common use for "small" devices because of the reduced amount of overhead (compared to IPv6, for example) and demands less energy to transmit data when compared to long range standards (UMTS, LTE or WiMax) [3].

For these reasons, with a client-server application design in mind, an additional functional element (the gateway (GW)) translates between both short and long range communication technologies and helps expending the boundaries of the current Internet. From an addressing perspective, these gateways are called Address Translation Gateways [18] due to their dual addressing function (IP and IEEE 802.15.4 in 6LoWPAN, for instance).

This paper focuses on the use of eHealth technologies in an IPv6 vehicular setting as a special V2I non-time-critical application. The operational scenario studied involves the use of eHealth devices, Electrocardiograph (ECG), Spirometer, Oximeter or Blood Glucose meter sending health-related measurements over Bluetooth to an IPv6-ready phone application. The phone is attached to an IPv6 Mobile Router (second part of the testbed). When the phone application (Android based) sends these measurements after user review and comments, to an application server in the IPv6 Internet, the Mobile Router ensures the right path is selected. Upon delivery, the gathered data is viewed remotely by the user's physician on his/her personal terminal.

The remainder of this paper is structured as follows. Section 2 describes the IPv6 communications requirements that apply to the M2M world. Section 3 presents the overall integrated platform and details its functional elements along with the considered scenario. Section 4 covers the default route configuration with an extension to Dynamic Host Configuration Protocol version 6 (DHCPv6) proposed at the Internet Engineering Task Force (IETF). Section 5 describes the hardware specifications and the integration process of the prototype used in experimentation. Section 6 covers the related work and positions our platform among state-of-the-art solutions. Section 7 concludes the paper and gives some envisaged perspectives for our platform.

2   M2M IPv6 Communications

As stated earlier, in the longer term, large-scale deployments of various M2M appliances will bring hundreds of millions of communicating devices to the currently deployed network. This perspective assumes that newly deployed devices will communicate in an unattended manner. In this scenario, the Internet Protocol family could glue all the parts of the heterogeneous wireless communication technologies used during the deployment, hence the importance of auto-configuration mechanisms (with no human intervention) of network parameters to build an end-to-end model from the application server to the endpoint. Two indivisible parts of the configuration process are studied below: addressing and routing.

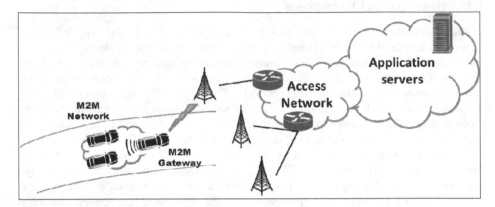

Fig. 1. M2M general system architecture. When the M2M gateway attaches to the network, the M2M gateway sets the PDN Gateway as its first hop towards the Internet and configures its IPv6 address using IPv6 stateless auto-configuration. An additional IPv6 prefix for the internal network is requested via DHCPv6 Prefix delegation.

2.1   Addressing

In order to configure a device with the necessary settings allowing it to communicate on a network, two types of mechanisms exist: stateful and stateless. The state here refers to the management information kept at the gateway level and the device. The configuration parameters usually include the address, mask, and a default route. DHCPv6 protocol falls within a stateful group since it maintains a database with all the assigned addresses to a specific device (leases file) at the DHCPv6 Server. Neighbor discovery protocol (NDP) on the other hand, which belongs to the stateless group, does not maintain such information: a Router provides a prefix to device and the device forms an address for itself without further assistance from other entities.

In the vehicular-eHealth scenario we are studying, IP devices are deployed in a vehicle equipped with a Gateway offering long-range connectivity. Hence auto-configuration mechanisms are needed. As depicted in Figure 1, the Gateway in addition to its egress interface address, requires a set of addresses (one or several prefixes) for the IP eHealth devices. The query is made through Prefix Delegation, an extension to the DHCPv6 protocol [23]. Basically, this extension allows the assignment of a set of prefixes to a Client. The DHCPv6 protocol is specified to work with Relay and Server entities several hopes away from the client, as described in this recent reference [24].

As vehicular gateways are designed for moving networks, Prefix Delegation for Network Mobility [25] has been specified and defines the behavior for the above DHCPv6 Prefix Delegation in the context of network mobility. In this work, focus is made on integration and the experimentations occur on table. Mobility scenarios could be part of future work.

2.2   Routing

In a vehicular network, routing must be set up in addition to assigning IPv6 addresses to the phone handling the eHealth devices. Discovering and configuring routes for large networks may quickly become a communication- and computing-intensive task, overcoming the capacity of the existing network. The concept of default route (gateway of last resort) provides partial resolution to this problem: it is sufficient for Gateway to hold a single default route (the IP address of the next hop) instead of detailed routes towards specific destinations. Default route auto-configuration mechanisms exist basically under two distinct forms. The first is Router Advertisement-based (the use of stateless address auto-configuration) and the second is a dynamic routing protocol such as OSPF [26]. Currently these two mechanisms are the only IETF mechanisms to assign a default route to an end node.

Whereas NDP address auto-configuration offers a default route to an end device, it does not offer a set of prefixes. Similarly, the DHCPv6 Prefix Delegation part of the stateful address auto-configuration does offer a set of addresses to the Gateway (in order to further deliver them to the IP eHealth devices) but does not offer a default route.

For a limited capacity device (a constrained vehicular Gateway, a Phone, or a constrained IP-eHealth device), it is advantageous to use a lightweight auto-configuration protocol offering both parameters:

- An IPv6 route to be used as a default route in the routing table of the Gateway.
- A set of IPv6 addresses, to be used for address auto-configuration on the IP eHealth devices on-board the vehicle.

3   Platform Integration

The objective of the platform described in this paper is to create a vehicular setting that integrates eHealth technology and improves current phone connectivity using next-generation communication capabilities. This section describes the functional elements involved in our architecture resulting from the integration phase both testbeds. The hardware specifications and the current state of the joint testbed are further detailed in the implementation section.

Figure 2 depicts the overall picture of the integrated testbed. The system includes 4 functional elements and 2 types of interactions (short and long-range).

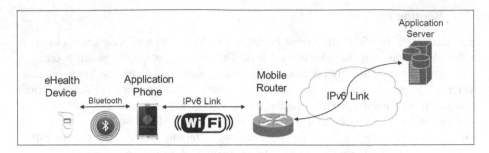

Fig. 2. Overall picture of the platform after integration. The eHealth devices communicate with the server through the phone application. The phone peers with the device over Bluetooth on one side, and attaches to the gateway over WiFi on the other. The gateway routes any traffic originated by the application to the PHR server in the infrastructure.

3.1 Functional Elements

In Figure 2, from left to right, the functional elements are as follows.

- **The eHealth Device** provides real time health-related measurements. These measurements can be of different nature such as blood glucose levels or oxygen saturation levels. Recorded data is sent over Bluetooth to another authorized peer and presented to the patient through a user interface.
- **The Application Phone** is in the middle of two different communication technologies. On one hand, short-range Bluetooth technology to communicate with M2M Devices, capture the eHealth data and present it to the patient and on the other hand, mid-range WiFi technology to send secure IPv6 packets to the server via the Gateway. The phone allows to process the gathered data before sending it to the server along with user comments, which is not possible with a standalone gateway.
- **The Mobile Router (MR)** provides IPv6 connectivity to in-vehicle devices and a default-route towards the server on the Internet. The gateway uses WiFi to advertise internal IPv6 prefix to the attached nodes. For the long-range communication technology (path towards the server), UMTS or LTE provide an IPv6 path from end to end. For testbed purposes, we demonstrate the concept over Ethernet (IEEE 802.3). The MR has a powerful CPU and provides some resource-demanding networking applications, not available to run on a limited battery power device like a smartphone. Besides, it is possible to request a higher Quality of Service upon network attachment for the MR that could be beneficial to the phone and other attached devices.
- **The Application Server** collects the data captured on patients and provides a web interface for doctors to support their diagnostic decisions. The software running on the server includes a web server accessed over a secure connection (over SSL) and a limited-access database server to gather the data issued by patients.

3.2   Operational Scenario

Vehicular networking and eHealth technologies are combined in the form of an ambulance equipped with special telemedicine devices that can record as well as transmit the patient's vital signs (body temperature, pulse rate, respiration rate, blood pressure) and critical physiological parameters (ECG, blood glucose levels, oxygen saturation levels) to the nearest hospital in order for the resident health professionals to optimally prepare the patient's admittance. This typical V2I scenario that is already possible with state-of-the-art technologies (IPv4 gateways) can be enhanced and tested in an IPv6 deployed architecture. This scenario could be applied to a situation where a road accident involving serious trauma is to be taken into consideration. The ambulance crew has in its disposition a set of handheld lightweight devices (as demonstrated in the prototyping section) that can transfer emergency data to the hospital. The objective in such a situation is to maximize clinical value through a limited set of measurements. All involved devices communicate via Bluetooth to an Android smart phone providing for IPv6 connectivity to the vehicular gateway that has reserved network resources to achieve certain QoS.

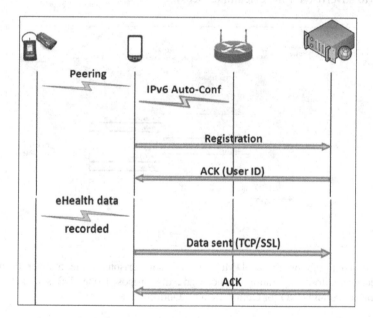

Fig. 3. Message exchange for the eHealth Operational Scenario. Vital signs recorded by the patient are sent to the expert for diagnosis.

However in an emergency situation (natural disaster, road accidents) where numerous vehicles of different functions (ambulances, fire brigade, police cars) are involved, the scenario could be enriched to accommodate for the optimum data transfer to the interested parties (health care provision, law enforcement) via V2V communications. This topic is out of scope of this paper.

4   Default Route Configuration with DHCPv6

As described in section 2, in order to configure in-vehicle devices we need to provide them with IPv6 prefixes requested from the infrastructure (PDN-GW) through DHCPv6 Prefix Delegation. In addition, the configuration of the attached gateway with an egress global address and a default route requires the use of NDP.

The proposal [27] depicted in the message exchange of Figure 4 shows the replacement of NDP by a DHCPv6 extension in the communications between the gateway and the infrastructure. The draft describes a new DHCPv6 option, Option Request Option (ORO) that allows to request, among other parameters, the default route. Figure 4 summarizes the extended message exchange performed by the vehicular Gateway and the DHCPv6 entities in the infrastructure. The original DHCPv6 protocol uses up to 10 messages in order for the gateway to obtain a set of addresses and a default route (that includes NDP interactions). In detail, the initial RS (Router Solicitation)/RA (Router Advertisement) offer the default route whereas the subsequent DHCP Solicit/Advertize/Request/Reply offer the set of addresses to the Gateway (to advertise for the eHealth devices).

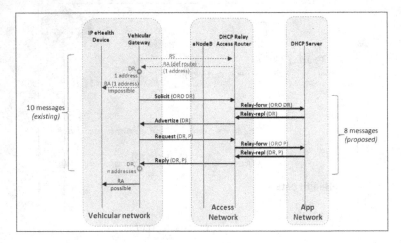

Fig. 4. Auto-configuration Protocol Messages. A comparison of the number of messages between current auto-configuration methods and the proposed one. DR stands for Default Route, P for prefix, and ORO for Option-Request Option.

Our proposal uses DHCPv6 messages only to provide the default route in addition to the set of addresses. The total number of messages of the earlier exchange is decreased from 10 to 8. The overall overhead due to control messages is reduced to optimize the bandwidth and the number of Round Trip Time (RTT) reduce. The practical gain depends on the quality of the link between the gateway and the infrastructure which cannot be measured in our testbed conditions.

The draft [27] details the operations executed by involved parties in the protocol. In a Solicit/Request packet a client lists the wanted options in the Option Request

Option (ORO), composed of a list of option codes. The DHCPv6 Server answers these packets with Advertise/Reply packets containing values for the options asked by the Client.

The relay receives the message from the client and forwards it to the server in a Relay-forward message. The server replies to the relay with an advertise/reply message encapsulated in a Relay-reply message. The content of this message is extracted by the relay and sent to the client.

In its DHCPv6 requests, the client sends a list of required options in the option request option (ORO). This option contains 3 mandatory fields: OPTION ORO, option-len and requested-option-code, followed by new option fields.

The proposed option is named here OPTION DEFAULT ROUTER LIST. It is possible to concatenate this value with several other existing requested-option-codes. The value of this code in this option is to be assigned. Obviously, this option needs to be understood by the server as well.

In the server side, the default router list option of DHCPv6 contains: OPTION DEFAULT ROUTER LIST, option-len, router-address, router-lifetime, lla len (link-layer address length) and optionally router link layer address. As this option contains a list, the pattern containing router address, router lifetime, lla len and optionally router link layer address can be repeated.

5   Prototype Implementation

This section describes technical aspects of the experimentation relating to testbed integration performed recently[1]. The high level goal is to demonstrate the capability of eHealth devices to communicate their specific data on the next-generation Internet from a vehicular setting. The underlying network communication protocols used were relying exclusively on IPv6. The application-layer protocols included, but were not limited to, HTTP and HTTPS.

5.1   Hardware Specification

Figure 5 depicts the M2M Gateway used in the experimentations. The Kerlink Wirma Road is an energy-efficient ARM926EJ-S platform provided with a 2.6.27 Linux kernel. In embedded computing field, the ARM926EJ-S processor is one of the most popular ARM processors, as it combines energy efficiency with enough CPU performance for most networking applications.

The M2M GW platform provides several communication capabilities. An integrated chipset provides only GSM/GPRS Cellular network service. An integrated WiFi module provides IEEE 802.11b/g connection. An integrated GPS module provides accurate geo-graphic coordinates. GPRS, WiFi and GPS antennas are unified in one vehicle roof antenna as depicted in Figure 5. In the front panel, an Ethernet

---

[1] At the time of writing, Authors present early results from the ongoing FP7 EXALTED (EXpAnding LTE for Devices) project. More details here: http://www.ict-exalted.eu

Hub and Serial connections (CAN, RS 232) are present. According to the manufacturer, 10% of the regional buses company in Paris (France) are equipped with this gateway. For testbed purposes, an additional NETGEAR Access Point (AP) is plugged into the Brick with a USB-Ethernet converter. Its purpose is to ease mobile phones attachment to the network advertised by the AP protected by a WEP Key.

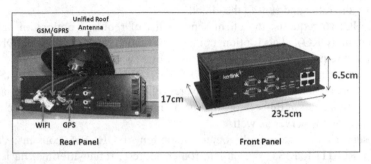

Fig. 5. Kerlink Wirma Road M2M Gateway. Factory settings propose M2M applications over IPv4-only networks. A kernel recompiling by cross-compilation has been performed to upgrade the capabilities of the platform in order to support next-generation protocols and include new drivers.

The eHealth devices (Figure 6) used for the testbed are manufactured by CardGuard [28] while the Android phone application is provided by Vidavo. The oxygen saturation level is measured by OxyPro, a wireless pulse oximeter. It provides for real time measurements and can be operated in continuous mode. It also provides for pulse monitoring. It displays oxygen saturation and pulse rate averages with the absolute maximum and minimum measurements.

The blood glucose and pressure measurement is performed by Easy2Check device. Blood glucose is measured with the use of an amperometric biosensor where fresh capillary blood is deposited. Its accuracy ranges from ±15mg/dL when glucose <75mg/dL to ±20% when glucose >75mg/dL. Accordingly for the pressure measurements the accuracy is ±3mmHg or ±2% of reading.

Self-check ECG offers 1 to 12 leads ECG events monitoring. It is intended for monitoring symptoms that may suggest abnormal heart function: skipped beats, palpitations, racing heart, irregular pulse, faintness, lightheadedness, or a history of arrhythmia. The recording period is set at 32 seconds while the bandwidth is 0.05 - 35 Hz for the 12 Leads and 0.4 - 35 Hz for the 1 Lead.

Spiro Pro is a spirometer that records Volume (Time and Volume) Flow curves according to international performance standards. It measures lung ventilatory functions during Forced Vital Capacity (FVC) tests. The recording lasts for 17 seconds and its accuracy for the FVC and FEV 1 is +5% or +0.1L. It is mostly used for asthma or COPD monitoring.

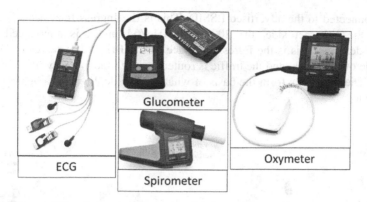

Fig. 6. Vidavo eHealth Devices. Different vital signs with different clinical value are observed. Captured data is sent over Bluetooth to the application.

A medical application is installed on an Android smart phone (IPv6-capable) which receives the vital signs from the portable monitoring devices via Bluetooth. The recorded data from the devices are transferred automatically (in the absence of the Mobile Router) through the smartphone via GPRS, Ethernet or WiFi to a designated web centre (over IPv4). The application provides a simple Electronic Health Record (EHR) for disease management and treatment and initiates patients' active involvement in healthcare. Analytically, it features browsing on the exams history, viewing of the recorded data, downloading of a diagnosis or advice from a doctor, comments addition and more. The final destination of these data is the EHR of the patient who uses the devices and it is resident in a dedicated server from where it is accessible for reviewing under secure credentials by the treating physicians.

5.2 Detailed Integration Process

Although the experimentation was performed in a laboratory setting, the hardware equipment is deployable in a vehicle as is: Kerlink's Wirma Road (IPv6 Gateway) is a low-consumption PC platform dedicated to vehicles, whereas eHealth devices are used by professionals for health periodic check-up and continuous monitoring. The kernel support of IPv6 and its associated extensions has been implemented in the gateway during the initial phase of the testbed integration. The overall architecture is summarized in Figure 7.

In the joint testbed, the M2M GW runs Router ADVertisement Daemon (radvd), version 1.8.5 compiled for ARM platforms and available for Debian distributions [29]. The radvd is configured to advertise at regular intervals or immediately on solicitations, two different prefixes for two different interfaces. On the Air Interface (AP), which is bridged to the Brick, the 2001:DB8:B:2::/64 prefix is advertised for the devices connected to the advertised ESSID. This is the Ingress Interface of the M2M GW. On the Ethernet side, the 2001:DB8:A:1::/64 prefix is announced for the connected devices. This is the Egress Interface of the Brick. The server is connected on this side of the Brick, and the traffic is routed through the gateway from one end to the other. These devices form the basis of what will be deployed in a vehicle such as an ambulance.

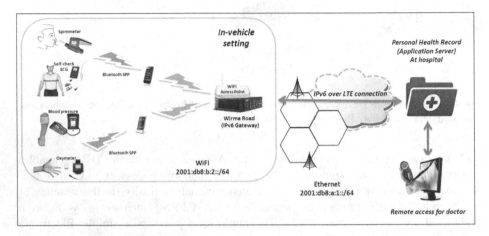

Fig. 7. eHalth and Vehicular testbeds integration. Future work includes replacing server-mobile router Ethernet link by LTE radio link.

As illustrated in Figure 7, on the vehicle side (ingress interface) two phone brands are used. (1) Samsung Galaxy 3 which runs Android 2.2 system. This phone is peered with the ECG and Spirometer devices over Bluetooth. (2) HTC Hero which runs Android 2.3 system. This phone is peered with the Glucometer and the oximeter over Bluetooth as well. Both phones are attached to the AP and configure IPv6 addresses on the 2001:DB8:B:2::/64 prefix. The devices are then used with the Vidavo Android Application that collects the data before sending it to the server over HTTPS along with a user comment (optional).

The server, which is located on the Internet side (Egress interface), configures an IPv6 address on the 2001:DB8:A:1::/64 prefix. The server is then ready to receive the data. The server application runs over Java (tomcat webserver) and includes a MySQL database, where the collected data is stored and organized per user ID. The physician can then issue a remote access to the server in order to observe the data as depicted in Figure 8. In order to observe these measurements (path from the viewer to the server), IPv4 and IPv6 access to the application server are possible.

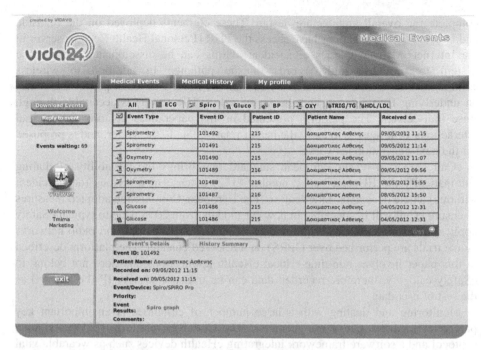

Fig. 8. Web Interface for remote viewer. The health care specialist will have access to the collected information along with patient comments.

6   Related Work

Generally speaking, eHealth protocol messages carry sensitive data and require integrity, confidentiality and availability. Privacy is also one major security concern. Pseudonymization of medical data is the typical solution that addresses this issue [19]. The proposed platform relies on an encrypted channel of communication originating from the application towards the server. Access to the information database (EHR) is reserved to the parties owning the right credentials.

The WEHealth platform [20] covers the topic of embedding eHealth systems in vehicular network. Basically, WEHealth provides eHealth service for medical needs on roads and enhances security and privacy by the use of the NOTICE framework (a secure and privacy-aware architecture for the notification of traffic incidents). The infrastructure of this proposal includes short-range communication capable sensor belts deployed along the road. The infrastructure in NOTICE uses embedded sensor belts on the road put at regular intervals (e.g., every mile or so). Each belt is composed of a collection of pressure sensors and a few small transceivers. The pressure sensors in each belt allow every message to be associated with a physical vehicle passing over the belt, eliminating the need to uniquely identify vehicles in order to interact with them. The sensor belts do not communicate with each other directly and rely on passing cars to carry and forward a message between adjacent belts. Check station belts (authentication centers) and pseudonyming proxies complete the overall architecture design. These elements deployed on the roadside and attached to Base Stations have access the PHR (Personal Health Record) server in the Internet. Medical queries or accident alarms can be disseminated through the system to provide health records of the patients. In addition to wireless communications with external sensor nodes on the road, WEHealth platform assumes an underlying IPv4 Internet and the server side (PHR server) is accessible through Base transceivers. The platform presented in this paper does not rely on external interactions with sensors to carry the health-related data to the server, and is proposed for the next-generation networks.

eCall [21] is a recent European standard that brings the possibility of dialing automatically the EU emergency number (112) in case of a serious road accident without vehicle occupants' intervention. The European Commission adopted measures to ensure eCall will be available in new car models from 2015. Due to typical eSafety applications stringent delay requirements, eCall is to operate only on radio networks (some trials are performed over GPRS) on a reserved channel. The platform described in this paper involves non-time-critical eHealth applications and does not belong to eSafety category, therefore recorded data can be transported over IP (best-effort) as the rest of user data.

Monitoring and dealing with a large number of casualties is an important key parameter to disaster response scenarios. The CodeBlue platform [22] pro-vides a protocol and a software framework integrating eHealth devices such as wearable vital sign sensors, handheld computers, and location-tracking tags to handle disaster response and emergency care scenarios. The prototype proposes to integrate device discovery, robust routing, traffic prioritization, security, and RF-based location tracking. In a disaster scenario, handheld computers carried by first responders receive and visualize multiple patients vital signs on the implemented application. Based on these observations, triage operation can help optimize the chances of survival. Along with these objectives, security and privacy are studied according to legal ramifications specific to the USA regulations. The platform presented in this paper does not focus on a disaster scenario and considers a more general use case. In addition, Internet next-generation communication standards are used (IPv6).

7   Conclusion and Future Work

The infrastructure of the Internet is continuously evolving to support new services. Intelligent Transportation Systems activities integrate the vision of future networks. The deployed applications should help to preserve lives and make transportation safer and efficient. eHealth, if supported by vehicular networks could be one of the applications improving vehicle passengers safety.

This paper describes the integration process of vehicular and eHealth testbeds. The vehicular network is designed to work over a fully deployed IPv6 network. eHealth testbed collects, stores and sends health-related measurements to a PHR Server located in the infrastructure where the results can be viewed by a doctor. Performed experimentation demonstrates the capability of eHealth specific data to be sent on the next-generation Internet from a vehicular setting. The underlying network communication protocols used were relying exclusively on IPv6. The application-layer protocols included, but were not limited to, HTTP and HTTPS. The hardware used in this configuration is deployable, as it is, in a vehicle.

Next steps ahead include quality and performance measurements. Actual in-vehicle integration and demonstration of cellular capabilities of the M2M GW are next. In the near future, a method for IPv6 Vehicle-to-Vehicle-to-Infrastructure (V2V2I) communications based on DHCPv6 and Neighbor Discovery extensions, as detailed in the Auto-configuration Protocol section will be described along with a set of experiment results.

Acknowledgement. This work has been performed in the framework of the ICT project ICT-258512 EXALTED, which is partly funded by the European Union. Authors would like to thank involved partners for the technical support. The authors would also like to thank, M. Mouton (internship 2011) for his implementation of the default router list with DHCPv6, A. Kaiser and S. Decremps, for their valuable support.

References

1. Introduction. In: Hartenstein, H., Laberteaux, K.P. (eds.) VANET: Vehicular Applications and Inter-Networking Technologies, ch. 1, pp. 1–19. John Wiley & Sons (2010)
2. Foh, K.-L.: Integrating Healthcare: The Role and Value of Mobile Operators in eHealth, GSM Association mHealth Programme (October 03, 2012), http://www.gsma.com/mobilefordevelopment/wp-content/uploads/2012/05/Role-and-Value-of-MNOs-in-eHealth1.pdf
3. Deploying Wireless Sensor Devices in Intelligent Transportation System Applications. In: Abdel-Rahim, A. (ed.) Intelligent Transportation Systems, ch. 6, pp. 143–168. InTech Design Team (2012)
4. Roberts, J.: The clean-slate approach to future Internet design: a survey of research initiatives. Annals of Telecommunications (Annales Des Télécommunications) 64(5-6), 271–276 (2009)
5. ETSI Intelligent Transport Systems (ITS) (May 07, 2012), http://etsi.org/WebSite/Technologies/IntelligentTransportSystems.aspx
6. Evans, D.: The Internet of Things, The Next Evolution of the Internet, Cisco IBSG (Internet Business Solutions Group) (October 03, 2012), http://www.slideshare.net/CiscoIBSG/internet-of-things-8470978
7. Raunio, B.: The Internet of things. A report from the November 5, 2009 seminar, SE:s Internet guide, nr. 16, English edition, Sweden (2009)
8. Heuser, L., Nochta, Z., Trunk, N.-C.: Towards the Internet of Things. In: ICT Shaping the World: A Scientific View, ch. 5. John Wiley & Sons (2008)
9. The IANA IPv4 Address Free Pool is Now Depleted, American Registry for Internet Numbers (ARIN) (October 03, 2012), https://www.arin.net/announcements/2011/20110203.html
10. World IPv6 Launch, The Internet Society (October 03, 2012), http://www.worldipv6launch.org/
11. Gustafson, D.H., Wyatt, J.C.: Evaluation of ehealth systems and services. British Medical Journal 328, 1150 (2004)

12. Pagliari, C., Sloan, D., Gregor, P., Sullivan, F., Detmer, D., Kahan, J.P., Oortwijn, W., MacGillivray, S.: What is eHealth (4): a scoping exercise to map the field. J. Med. Internet Res. 7(1), e9 (2005)
13. Toor, Y., Muhlethaler, P., Laouiti, A.: Vehicle Ad Hoc networks: applications and related technical issues. IEEE Communications Surveys & Tutorials 10(3), 74–88 (2008)
14. Stancil, D.D., Bai, F., Cheng, L.: Communication systems for Car-2-X Networks. In: Vehicular Networking, Automotive Applications and Beyond, ch. 3, pp. 45–81. Wiley (2010)
15. Geographic addressing and routing for vehicular communications (GeoNet), FP7 ICT (October 03, 2012), http://www.geonet-project.eu/?pageid=9
16. 3GPP Long Term Evolution (October 03), http://ipv6.com/articles/wireless/3GPP-Long-Term-Evolution.htm
17. Gosse, K., et al.: Standardization of vehicle-to-Infrastructure Communication. In: Vehicular Networking, Automotive Applications and Beyond, ch. 8, pp. 171–201. Wiley (2010)
18. Mulligan, G.: The 6LoWPAN architecture. In: Proceeding of EmNets 2007, Cork, Ireland (2007)
19. Slamanig, D., Stingl, C.: Privacy aspects of ehealth. In: Third International Conference on Availability, Reliability and Security (ARES), pp. 1226–1233 (2008)
20. Yan, G., Wang, Y., Weigle, M.C., Olariu, S., Ibrahim, K.: WEHealth: A Secure and Privacy Preserving eHealth Using NOTICE. In: Proceedings of the International Conference on Wireless Access in Vehicular Environments (WAVE), Dearborn, MI (December 2008)
21. eSafety: eCall j emergency call for car accident Europa-Information Society (October 03, 2012), http://ec.europa.eu/information_society/activities/esafety/ecall/index_en.htm
22. Lorincz, K., Malan, D.J., Fulford-Jones, T.R.F., Nawoj, A., Clavel, A., Shnayder, V., Mainland, G., Welsh, M., Moulton, S.: Sensor networks for emergency response: challenges and opportunities. IEEE Pervasive Computing 3(4), 16–23 (2004)
23. Troan, O., Droms, R.: IPv6 Prefix Options for Dynamic Host Configuration Protocol (DHCP) version 6. IETF (2003)
24. Yeh, L., Tsou, T., Boucadair, M., Schoenwaelder, J., Hu, J.: Prefix Pool Option for DHCPv6 Relay Agents on Provider Edge Routers. IETF (Internet Draft), draft-yeh-dhc-dhcpv6-prefix-pool-opt-05 (2011)
25. Droms, R., Thubert, P., Dupont, F., Haddad, W., Bernardos, C.: Request for Comments: 6276, DHCPv6 Prefix Delegation for Network Mobility (NEMO). IETF (2011)
26. Lindem, A., Arkko, J.: OSPFv3 Auto-Configuration. IETF (Internet Draft), draft-acee-ospf-ospv3-autoconfig-00 (2011)
27. Petrescu, A., Janneteau, C., Mouton, M.: Default Router List Option for DHCPv6 (DRLO). IETF (Internet-Draft), draft-mouton-mif-dhcpv6-drlo-01 (2012)
28. Card Guard Products & Technologies (October 03, 2012), http://www.cardguard.com/cardguard
29. Linux IPv6 Router Advertisement Daemon (radvd) (October 03, 2012), http://www.litech.org/radvd/

Multimedia Chair Design for Improving the Experience of Hospital Stay for Children with Cancer: The Escape

Wout Kregting and Wei Chen

Department of Industrial Design, Eindhoven University of Technology,
Den Dolech 2, 5612 AZ, Eindhoven, The Netherlands
w.j.w.kregting@student.tue.nl, wjwkregting@gmail.com,
w.chen@tue.nl

Abstract. Children with cancer staying in isolation rooms at hospitals often feel lonely and disconnected from their family and friends. In this paper, we present the design and development of the Escape, which is a chair embedded with multimedia networks. The chair is designed and developed to a product ready for hospital use, in collaboration with VanBerlo Design, Catharina Hospital, Webchair, and MaraThOON Foundation of the Netherlands, for improving these children's experience of their hospital stay and enhancing their bonding with the outside world. The paper describes the user centered design process, multimedia technology integration, implementation and production of the ambient media system.

Keywords: ambient media, entertainment, children with cancer, multimedia chair, ambient intelligence.

1 Introduction

In the Netherlands, about 500 children are confronted with cancer every year and in the United States in 2007, approximately 10,400 children under age 15 were diagnosed with cancer and about 1,545 children will die from the disease [1]. These children's carefree life suddenly turns into a life in which they have to spend much time in the isolation rooms at hospital. They can't do the things they used to do and they can't attend school. They see their friends less and less frequently. Therefore, to improve their experience of the hospital stay and enhance their bonding with the outside world, we proposed and developed a chair embedded with multimedia networks called 'Escape', in collaboration with VanBerlo Design, Catharina Hospital, Webchair, and MaraThOON Foundation of the Netherlands.

Together with the development of the ambient intelligence concept [2], recent advances in sensor and multimedia networking technologies [3-5] enable the creation of a new generation of healthcare systems with smart environments. Ambient media and systems cover a wide range of applications, including healthcare, sports, work, entertainment, etc. For example, to improve the comfort of passengers by an adaptive entertainment system, non-invasive sensors for heart rate monitoring were embedded in the aircraft passenger seat, enabling the emotion model manager to choose the proper music in the database for reducing the stress of the passenger [6]. Another

C.T. Angelis, D. Fotiadis, and A.T. Tzallas (Eds.): AMBI-SYS 2013, LNICST 118, pp. 81–90, 2013.
© Institute for Computer Sciences, Social Informatics and Telecommunications Engineering 2013

example is to support economy class passengers to sleep well during a long haul flight. The sleeping posture of a passenger is detected by pressure sensors embedded in the aircraft seat, enabling the smart seat to provide support to the passenger [7, 8]. A user friendly EEG headset has been designed to enhance people's wellbeing based on bio-feedback[9]. For the elderly, unobtrusive sensor technologies for sleeping patterns [10] and health status of people living alone at home [11] have been reported. Intelligent designs for critically ill babies at hospitals have been developed in user centered approaches, such as vital signs monitoring for neonates [12-15], data transmission [16], a power supply for neonatal monitoring [17], neonatal behavioral state detection based on facial expression analysis [18], and a device to support cardiopulmonary resuscitation of neonates [19]. To increase the quality of life of children with bone marrow transplantation, the University Hospital Essen offers isolation rooms with multimedia facilities, such as a flat-screen TV, PlayStation 3 with Move, WebChair, Philips ambient light, etc..

In this paper, we present the design and development of the Escape, which is a chair embedded with multimedia networks. Multidisciplinary knowledge and collaboration are involved throughout the user centered design process. The comfort chair is designed with integration of the techniques and research from medical science and practice, ergonomics, materials, and multimedia technologies. The comfort chair is specially designed for children with cancer staying at hospitals. Our chair with multi-media functions will help them to stay connected and actively communicate with their family and friends. We have transferred the design from a full-scale prototype to a real product. The intelligent multimedia chair has been exhibited during the Dutch Design Week 2012 and by the end of the year the chair will be used in the wards of Catherina hospital in the Netherlands.

2   Design Process and Design Concept

2.1   Design Process

The design process to create the multimedia entertainment chair is shown in Fig. 1. In each phase of the process, iterations were carried out.

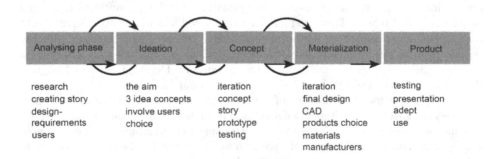

Fig. 1. Design process

The first phase is the analyzing phase. In this phase is knowledge gained from user study and background information will be translated into values and requirements for the design.

Sheldon [20] compiled a list of values that are important to humans. Which values are most important for the target group? The age of children with cancer can be range from 0 till 18 years old, but it is impossible the design a good product that fits all age-groups. Thus the age group of 8 -15 was chosen to design for. The children in this group are late elementary school to middle high school. They are usually familiar with multimedia systems for games or entertainments. Through interviews with doctors, healthy children and parents, the following values are found very important:

- *Relatedness;* contact with family and friends
- *Pleasure stimulation;* entertainment
- *Security;* safe feeling
- *Privacy;* an own place in a isolation room full of windows

Next to the value, design requirements are gained by age group research, trend research, and interviewing people at the Catharina hospital in the Netherlands, including doctors, technical employees, patients and isolation ward. The requirements are listed below:

General requirements

- The chair is suitable for children with cancer (weaker and less physically healthy than normal children
- The target group of the comfort chair is 8 till 15 years
- In the chair the nurses and the doctors are able to do the same tests as in the hospital bed
- The chair is cleanable by the standards of the isolation ward of the Catharina Hospital in the Netherlands
- The chair is mobile
- The chair fits to a door: length 2000mm, width 1000mm
- The chair meets the safety requirements of hospitals

Design and user aspects

- The chair is an eye catcher
- The chair fits in a hospital environment
- The design is understood by the user
- The chair has a safe look and feel
- The chair offers communication to friends, family and school
- The chair offers privacy for the patients
- The patient is visible for the doctors while using the chair (the doctors has to monitor the patients)
- The chair is safe for the user
- The user has influence on the environment (Cancer patients are dependent on their environments, so influence on the environment enables their feeling of having some control)

Technical requirements

- The electronics in the chair works with the European 220 -240 Volts sockets
- The chair includes entertainment with a CE hallmark
- The multimedia system provides video, music, games, and internet access
- The multimedia system should be compatible with the hospital environments
- The system should be easy to clean for hygiene purposes

After formulating the requirements and the values, the aim is important. The aim has a strong connection with the users. The users are the patients in the hospital. But these patients are almost the same as normal kids. During the user-research the focus was on healthy children, because the sick children want to be like the healthy children. And the healthy children are kids who go to school, play with their friends, communicate through social media etc. Concluding, the aim is a chair that fulfills the wishes of healthy children.

And then the ideation starts with ideas and sketches. Fig. 2 shows some sketches of ideas. During this phase the results of the analyzing phase are continuously used. The results of this phase were three idea-concepts. The chosen idea-concept focused on privacy, safe feeling, full entertainment and a patient's own place.

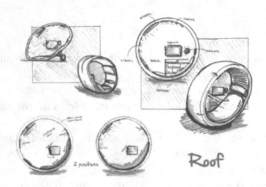

Fig. 2. Sketches of ideas

After the idea-concept choice, first iteration starts. Start from zero with this idea-concept and bring it to concept level. This means, adding materials, colors, ergonomics, multimedia details etc. To test the concept a scale model is made.

The fourth step is materialization. During this step, feedback from the previous phases has to be analyzed and serve as inputs for the new iteration. In this phase choices have to be made, nothing can be uncertain anymore. After this phase the design is producible by manufactures.

2.2   Design Concept

The design concept is to create a personal multimedia system for the patients, which is an escape from the isolation room, escape from the hospital, and escape from cancer. This place adapts to the user and creates a safe feeling. The technologies help the patient stay connected and provide entertainment options.

The basic idea is to create for the patient their own place in a chair, like a small room. This concept offers privacy, because the roof of the patient is covered, like sitting in an arcade-hall device. The person playing on the arcade unit game is totally in the game and feels like he has privacy, and in the meanwhile still a lot of people can see the person. The form of a circle came up by analyzing the patients during the analyzing phase. The patients live in a horrible circle of life. This design offers an Escape from the isolated life in a hospital ward through a circle shape chair.

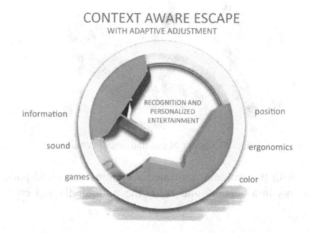

Fig. 3. Design concept of a context aware multimedia chair

We envision a context aware multimedia chair as shown in Fig. 3. The chair will recognize the patient when he or she enters the chair. The chair will automatically change its preferences to the patient (sitting position, sound, ergonomics, lights etc.). The chair can give the patient information about its situation/disease. The chair can also adapt to the mood of the patient, for example cheer the patient up with entertainment suggestions.

The hard part of being a designer is to translate an idea-concept to a product. Based on the hardware availability and the requirements (e.g. hygiene, safety, etc.), only products with a CE mark will be integrated in the design.

Fig. 4 illustrates the concept of the multimedia chair. It is in a circled shape to provide a private and cozy feeling. The product concept needs a more defined multimedia and the experience we want to create. The multimedia technologies from WebChair BV (www.webchair.com) are integrated in the concept. With WebChair software and hardware, patients can communicate with their friends, family and school by using an all-in-one PC or tablet. The concept also consists of social media and web browsing by an Internet connection, Gameconsole (PlayStation 3) with online function to play games alone or with friends (multiplayer), and a big screen with stereo sound system for the great entertainment experience. In addition, an adjustable light strip is included to offer the patient some control in the environments. The chair is rotatable with flexible sitting positions, such as an active position for schoolwork etc., middle position for web browsing, gaming etc. and relaxation position for movies, sleeping etc. Medical casters are used for moving the chair to other locations if necessary.

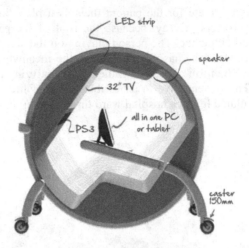

Fig. 4. Concept of the multimedia chair

By the design with the ambient multimedia systems, the child patient will forget that they are patients in a hospital and enjoy the multimedia and entertainment as a healthy child.

3   Prototype

To test this concept a prototype was made as shown in Fig. 5. This prototype is to see how the ergonomics are in this circle shaped chair, the feeling and how big it actually is.

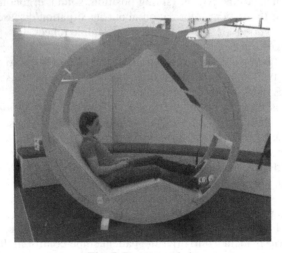

Fig. 5. Prototype chair

The prototype was tested with 40 people. The most important part was the sitting position. Can a person sit well the circle of the "Escape". The ergonomics were measured, but in reality it's always different. Overall the 1:1 model/prototype sits surprisingly well (especially for a wooden seat), but for people under the 1.70 has some problem with the seat length. Also the 1:1 model misses the lumbar and head support. This is necessary to sit for a longer time in the chair. The entertainment is on a nice distance from your body. With the overhead cover the users have the feeling that they have privacy. But still, the people around the chair can see the user. This is a very important part of the concept. Feeling privacy is important, but it is also important that the doctors can see the patient true the glass of the isolation room. And that the doctor can do checks while the patient is in the chair.

4   Product

After the materialization phase as described in Section 2, it is possible to produce the product. Figure 6 present the final design of the ambient multimedia chair - Escape.

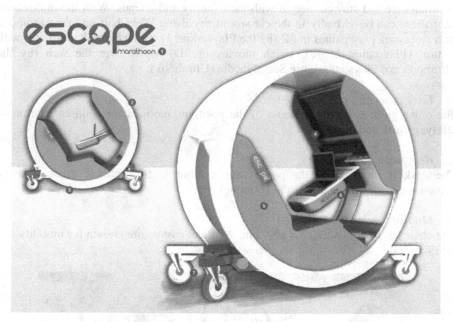

Fig. 6. Escape render with numbers

The key features of Escape is indicated on Fig. 6. They are the Logo, adjustable lamp, rotation and multi-sitting position, Multimedia networks for entertainment, easy clean and comfortable textile, removable desk, medical casters for mobility and fixation.

1. Logo
The escape is an iconic designed chair. The silhouette of the chair is represented within the Logo.

2.   Adjustable lamp
This lamp is shown on this picture. But with this lamp the user has the possibility to adjust the color of the space around him/her. With this function, the patient feels like he or she has influence on the environment.

3.   Rotation and multi-sitting position
The entire circle is rotatable; hence the chair can be adjusted to three stand/positions. Active position for schoolwork etc., middle position for web browsing, gaming etc. and relax position for movies, sleeping etc. The circle is rotatable because of the wheels placed on the steel construction at the outside of the chair.

4.   Multimedia networks for entertainment
The escape has multimedia networks embedded for entertainment including a 32-inch 3D TV (Philips 32PFL6007), Playstation 3 with Move, Soundbar (Samsung HW-E350), Ultrabook (ACER ASPIRE S5) and lighting (Philips Living Colors). The multimedia networks have access to Internet so that children with cancer can communicate and stay connected with their family and friends. With the multimedia the patient can be virtually in the classroom (by using WebChair and the Ultrabook with webcam), play games in 3D (by the Playstation 3) with a controller but also with motion (Playstation Move), watch movies in 3D, brows over the web (by the Ultrabook and Playstation), use Social media (Ultrabook).

5.   Easy clean and comfortable textile
The color green is chosen because of the positive emotions for children: Harmony, safety, growth and comfort.

6.   Removable desk
The desk is included so the patient has a table to for example draw or make homework and also a place for the Ultrabook.

7.   Mobility and safe fixation
The chair has to be mobile, but also safe. Medical casters are chosen for mobility and safe fixation.

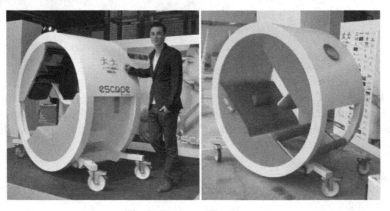

Fig. 7. Product - The Escape

Fig. 7. shows the actual product to be used in the Catharina Hospital of Netherlands. The product has been exhibited in the Dutch Design Week in Eindhoven Oct. 2012.

5   Future Work

Further research and design will be conducted to design and implement the context aware multimedia chair to provide the adaptive personal entertainment experience. User research will also be carried out in hospitals to study the user experience with the proposed intelligent chair. The feedback from evaluations will be used as inputs for the design improvement.

6   Conclusion

Children with cancer staying in isolation rooms at hospitals often feel lonely and disconnected from their family and friends. In this paper, we present the design and development of the Escape, which is a chair embedded with multimedia networks. The chair is designed and developed to a product ready for hospital use, in collaboration with VanBerlo Design, Catharina Hospital, Webchair, and MaraThOON Foundation of the Netherlands, for improving these children's experience of their hospital stay and enhancing their bonding with the outside world.

Acknowledgment. The design process and manufacturing of the escape would not have been possible without the support and endless effort of a number of individuals. The authors are particularly grateful to Thomas Paulen and Prof. Ad van Berlo from VanBerlo Design, Graham Smith from Webchair, Dr. Natasja Dors, Dr. Edwin Knots and Dr. Vera Lagerburg from the Catharina Hospital Eindhoven, and Prof. dr. Sidarto Bambang Oetomo from Eindhoven University of Technology for their information, feedback and advising support. We thank Dr. Oliver Basu from the University Hospital Essen in Germany for hosting our visit to the hospital's high-tech isolation wards. We are very grateful to Harry-Anton Bloem from Foundation MaraThOON Netherlands for the advising and financial support.

References

[1] Childhood cancers, National Cancer Institute, http://www.cancer.gov/cancertopics/factsheet/Sites-Types/childhood
[2] Aarts, E.H.L., Encarnação, J.L.: True visions: The emergence of ambient intelligence, 2nd edn. Springer (2008)
[3] Tao, X.: Wearable electronics and photonics. Woodhead (2005)
[4] Yang, G., Yacoub, M.: Body sensor networks. Springer-Verlag New York Inc. (2006)
[5] Hwang, J.-N.: Multimedia Networking: From Theory to Practice. Cambridge University Press (2009)

[6] Liu, H., et al.: LsM: A New Location and Emotion Aware Web-based Interactive Music System. Presented at the Proceedings of IEEE International Conference on Consumer Electronics (ICCE 2010), Piscataway, NJ (2010)

[7] Tan, C., et al.: Sleeping Posture Analysis of Economy Class Aircraft Seat. In: World Congress on Engineering, London, U.K., pp. 532–535 (2009)

[8] Tan, C., et al.: Adaptive Framework and User Preference Modeling for Economy Class Aircraft Passenger Seat. In: Third UKSim European Symposium on Computer Modeling and Simulation, Athens, Greece, pp. 66–69 (2009)

[9] van Aart, J., et al.: EEG headset for neurofeedback therapy: enabling easy use in the home environment. In: International Conference on Bio-inspired Signals and Systems, pp. 23–30 (2008)

[10] Adami, A., et al.: Unobtrusive monitoring of sleep patterns. In: 25th Annual International Conference of the IEEE EMBS, pp. 1360–1363 (2003)

[11] Kaushik, A., Celler, B.: Characterization of PIR detector for monitoring occupancy patterns and functional health status of elderly people living alone at home. Technology and Health Care 15, 273–288 (2007)

[12] Bouwstra, S., et al.: Smart Jacket Design for Neonatal Monitoring with Wearable Sensors. In: Body Sensor Networks (BSN 2009), Berkeley, USA, pp. 162–167 (2009)

[13] Chen, W., et al.: Non-invasive blood oxygen saturation monitoring for neonates using reflectance pulse oximeter. Presented at the Design, Automation and Test in Europe - Conference and Exhibition 2010 (DATE 2010), Dresden, Germany (2010)

[14] Chen, W., et al.: Monitoring Body Temperature of Newborn Infants at Neonatal Intensive Care Units Using Wearable Sensors. To be Presented at the Fifth International Conference on Body Area Networks (BodyNets 2010), Corfu Island, Greece (2010)

[15] Potuzakova, D., et al.: Innovative Design for Monitoring of Neonates Using Reflectance Pulse Oximeter. In: 2011 7th International Conference on Intelligent Environments (IE), pp. 200–205 (2011)

[16] Chen, W., et al.: Wireless transmission design for health monitoring at neonatal intensive care units. Presented at the 2nd International Symposium on Applied Sciences in Biomedical and Communication Technologies (ISABEL 2009), Bratislava, Slovak Republic (2009)

[17] Chen, W., et al.: A design of power supply for neonatal monitoring with wearable sensors. Journal of Ambient Intelligence and Smart Environments 1, 185–196 (2009)

[18] Hazelhoff, L., Han, J., Bambang-Oetomo, S., de With, P.H.N.: Behavioral State Detection of Newborns Based on Facial Expression Analysis. In: Blanc-Talon, J., Philips, W., Popescu, D., Scheunders, P. (eds.) ACIVS 2009. LNCS, vol. 5807, pp. 698–709. Springer, Heidelberg (2009)

[19] Chen, W., et al.: Rhythm of Life Aid (ROLA) – An Integrated Sensor System for Supporting Medical Staff during Cardiopulmonary Resuscitation (CPR) of Newborn Infants. IEEE Transactions on Information Technology in Biomedicine 14, 1468–1474 (2010)

[20] Sheldon, K., et al.: What Is Satisfying About Satisfying Events? - Testing 10 Candidate Psychological Needs. Journal of Personality and Social Psychology 80, 325–339 (2001)

Devices and Wireless Interface Control in Vehicular Communications: An Autonomous Approach

Michelle Wetterwald and Christian Bonnet

EURECOM, Campus SophiaTech,
450 route des Chappes, 06410 Biot, France
{Michelle.Wetterwald,Christian.Bonnet}@eurecom.fr

Abstract. During recent years, mobile communications have reached every aspect of our modern life. Multimode wireless terminals are about to be introduced in our vehicles, giving them the capability to communicate through different networks. However, it is hardly possible for the car device to control efficiently and adapt dynamically its connectivity according to its environment. The objective of this paper is to present the concept of an innovative technological framework for the autonomous control of multimode terminals in heterogeneous and non-federated wireless environments. The aim is to enable a self-configuring terminal to connect to independent networks, while respecting its applications requirements. The target scheme implies a strong level of abstraction and cross-layer design, taking into account constraints based on heterogeneous wireless systems, autonomous architectures and enabling generic services such as a smart access network selection. This scheme applies to the mobile terminal only, with mechanisms independent of the network infrastructure. The paper analyses how existing technologies are enhanced and combined with new features to achieve this objective and gives a description of the overall concept. A simulated model is used to assess the validity of the proposed framework, together with applications to real systems, highlighting the key benefits of the concept.

Keywords: Heterogeneous networks, wireless access selection, intelligent transport applications, MIH.

1 Introduction

In the recent years, mobile communications have been evolving and growing very fast, together with an exponential use of the Internet for all sorts of applications such as voice calls, video streaming or Mobile TV. Multimode terminals, capable to connect in heterogeneous networks have been introduced in every aspect of our modern lives and are now almost ready to be deployed in our vehicles, where they will provide additional safety, traffic efficiency and entertainment. One of the challenges to be addressed by these new systems, also called On-Board Units (OBUs), is the choice of the optimal access network according to the requirements and constraints of the executing

C.T. Angelis, D. Fotiadis, and A.T. Tzallas (Eds.): AMBI-SYS 2013, LNICST 118, pp. 91–103, 2013.
© Institute for Computer Sciences, Social Informatics and Telecommunications Engineering 2013

applications. Currently, the software installed in smartphones prioritizes a Wi-Fi hotspot when one is detected, transferring all the data traffic on this access. When no Wi-Fi is available, the data traffic is transferred through the cellular network. This may lead to odd or unwanted behaviours. When it comes to OBUs, the constrained environment generates an additional level of complexity. Moreover, the OBU environment may rapidly change, especially due to the vehicle mobility, which implies a dynamic and autonomous adaptation of the device connectivity. It then becomes necessary to fine-tune dynamically the OBU connectivity on one or several of its network accesses according to the user's preferences or the needs of its applications. The current binomial and static solution is thus expected to become rapidly too limited and simplistic compared to the connectivity constraints foreseen in the near future, preventing safety applications which require very low latency to execute as initially planned. Techniques exist that partially address these requirements. First are the Media Independent Handover (MIH) services which provide mechanisms to handle multimode terminals when roaming across heterogeneous networks. Secondly, a new entity, the Connection Manager (CMGR) has been introduced to collect information about the device environment and apply algorithms optimizing the access network selection decision. A third technique comes from autonomous systems, which execute intelligent control loops, providing the ability to cope and adapt dynamically to unexpected situations according to decision policies. However, none of these techniques is able to provide a full solution by itself and efficiently take care of the diverse hardware devices located in the terminal. Our objective is thus to integrate them in a single framework which will provide the future systems with a flexible and optimized control of their multimode operation.

This paper is organised as follows. Section 2 exposes the challenge faced to connect efficiently and dynamically the vehicular devices and introduces the existing techniques which partially solve the issue: MIH services, access network selection and autonomous systems. Section 3 proposes an active and integrated framework which provides an intelligent control of the mobile terminal connectivity. It explains how this framework manages its various hardware devices and is organized to select autonomously the best suited access network. This is followed by an evaluation of the framework in section 4, together with its main results. The document is closed in Section 5 by a summary of the main contributions and the direction taken for future research.

2   Reference Technologies and Challenges

The section starts with an introduction of the specific challenges faced by vehicular communications. Then it presents existing technologies which partially address the issue of a dynamic and reliable adaptation of the wireless connectivity to heterogeneous access networks.

2.1   Vehicular Communications

A whole set of new technologies and applications are being designed [1] to enhance the quality of our travelling experience. This new domain constitutes a typical application case since car devices or OBUS can connect to at least three access technologies, including a specific wireless access derived from the Wi-Fi, also called the ITS (Intelligent Transport Systems) G5 technology, while they additionally receive information from the positioning system in the vehicle. The ITS architecture considers a varied set of devices: handheld terminals, cars, trucks, public vehicles and buses, but also traffic lights, variable message signs, traffic monitoring centres, etc. Accordingly, the new applications imply new constraints on the communications sub-system. Road safety applications developed to prevent car crashes require very low latency communications between the vehicles, achievable mainly with the ITS G5 access in V2V (Vehicle to Vehicle) mode. On the other hand, entertainment applications may require large bandwidths which can be obtained only with Wi-Fi or LTE (Long Term Evolution) cellular networks. As a consequence, the selection of the access network to be used depends not only on the radio signal level, but also on the application requirements and on other system parameters. Currently, the same application always uses the same type of access technology, whatever the context of the ITS Station. The terminal being multimode, each technology or modem requires the development of extensions to the control software in addition to the specific device drivers, which allows very little flexibility when moving between different environments. The ITS world is thus a typical case where a smart access technology selection algorithm, coupled with a strong level of abstraction for the monitoring and control of the different access technologies and mobile devices is required.

2.2   Media Independent Services

Operating multimode devices in heterogeneous networks can become very complex if each access technology has to be addressed directly and separately by the networking entities. To cope with this issue when executing access network handover, the IEEE 802.21 standard proposes three different Media Independent Services [2]. They offer to the upper layer management protocols some abstracted triggers, information acquisition and the tools needed to perform the handovers. The Event Service (MIES) provides the framework needed to manage the network events, and to report the dynamic status of the different links. The Command Service (MICS) allows controlling the links behaviour while the Information Service (MIIS) distributes the topology-related information and policies from a repository located in the network. A cross-layer architecture is defined where the MIH Function (MIHF), pictured in Figure 1, acts as a relay between *(i)* the media-specific Link layer entities connected by the MIH_LINK_SAP (Service Access Point) and *(ii)* the media-agnostic upper layer entities, or MIH-Users, connected over the MIH_SAP. The MIHF also handles the protocol that runs between the different network nodes to synchronize the MIH operations. This protocol provides rules for peer communications between the MIHF modules located in the different nodes and operates through the MIH_NET_SAP, using either Layer2 or Layer3 transport, according to the access network.

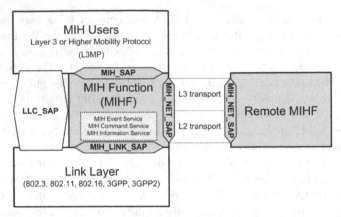

Fig. 1. Reference Model for Media Independent Handover

Currently, the IEEE 802.21 standard provides valuable mechanisms to control the network interfaces of a multimode terminal in a Media Independent and abstracted way. However, it involves several strong limitations. It only enables handover services and addresses exclusively network interfaces, ignoring the other devices present in the terminal which may reveal useful to control its connectivity. It thus offers the possibility to be developed to support an extended set of services and devices. This extension will be a main axis for the design of our solution.

2.3   Access Network Selection in Multimode Terminals

A research in literature on heterogeneous wireless network selection returns many studies and surveys for vertical handover management and optimization algorithms. A vast majority of them take the terminal point of view, optimizing network access selection in conjunction with mobility mechanisms. The main steps of the decision procedure are the input collection and the execution of a selection algorithm.

As explained in [3], the first step of the decision process consists in the collection of the appropriate information, according to a pre-defined list of criteria or attributes. In this survey, the attributes considered are all available from local resources, giving more importance to the user perspective: received signal strength, network connection time, available bandwidth, power consumption, monetary cost, security, and user's preferences. The authors in [4] have the objective to optimize the performance of the system by selecting the best interface for a generic file download service. The decision is made locally to avoid any impact on the network, hiding from the application the complexity of spreading traffic over different access networks. The selection is performed using attributes related to the user context, QoS and mobility. Some information may also be provided by entities in the network, such as the MIIS or the ANDSF (Access Network Discovery and Selection Function) [5]. The latter contains the data management and control functionality necessary for providing network discovery and selection assistance data to the MT as per operators' policy.

When these inputs have been collected, a selection algorithm is executed. Algorithms range from simple comparisons where the best signal quality is chosen, to more complex ones which smartly combine the additional parameters from the end user, the application or the network context. The authors of [3] provide a survey of classical decision strategies in 4th Generation networks, classifying them based on the decision criteria. They show that the preferred input is usually the RSS (Received Signal Strength), sometimes combined with bandwidth information. Cost functions are more complex and combined algorithms the most reliable, but at the cost of larger handover delays. [6] analyses and classifies the different existing strategies, including user-centric strategies, taking into account user preferences in terms of cost and QoS, or strategies resolving a Multi-Attribute Decision Making (MADM) problem. The paper surveys well-known methods such as SAW (Simple Additive Weighting), TOPSIS (Technique for Order Preference by Similarity to Ideal Solution) or WP (Weighted Products). [7] defines a method based on a Markov Decision Process, using a link reward associated with the QoS achieved by the mobile connection and evaluated against the cost of handover signalling. The results show better handover performance than more classical methods, but the converging time of the algorithm is of the order of magnitude of minutes. Moreover, most of the proposed algorithms require a continuous execution and thus consume a lot of processing power. This is not convenient in a mobile device with limited power resources.

2.4   Autonomic Systems

Other conception studies of future architectures introduce a totally new cognitive plane, where the environment is sensed and observed, leading to the acquisition of knowledge which is exploited in a novel capability of self-management [8]. These Autonomous Systems (AS) are adaptable to cope with unexpected situations or dynamic changes occurring in their environment. They are in continuous variation at all levels, whether it be data, environment or goals. The self-management is performed primarily according to some internal policies and without requiring actions from a human user. The system operates by undertaking intelligent control loops [9]. It senses its operating environment, works with models that analyse its own behaviour in that environment, and, based on existing policies and learned knowledge, derives the appropriate actions to adapt and change the environment, its own state or its behaviour.

The AS architecture is structured according to a decision hierarchy and coordinated by an Orchestration Autonomic Manager (OAM). The OAM is assisted by a Manual Manager (or human user) and lower level Autonomic Managers. In their turn, they monitor and control the Managed Resources through a so-called Manageability Interface. A basic and shared knowledge source is installed at setup and further enhanced by self-learning in an evolutionary process through progressive steps. These concepts are introduced mostly in large computing systems and in a very basic and semi-empirical way in the existing CMGR implementations, to decide on which access network the mobile should connect. By mirroring the self-management architectures currently defined at network level, it sounds interesting to make an analogy and apply the same concept to the self-configuration of the MT, more particularly to the coordination of the different technologies involved in the solution to our problem.

3 Extending the Media Independent Services

Because the decision between networks operated independently has to be taken by the control entities in the car device, the main and innovative approach proposed here is to modify only the mobile terminal, leaving the network totally unaffected. Connectivity has to be maintained efficiently while remaining transparent to the applications. The system will also capitalize on an extension of the abstraction model introduced in the MIH standard.

3.1 The Connectivity Control Framework

According to these objectives, a layered system, the Connectivity Control Framework (CCF) pictured in Figure 2, has been designed. Some of the components, shown in the figure with hatched blocks, are present in existing terminals and remain unchanged. They include the applications, the Networking Services (NS, e.g., existing handover, security mechanisms or network statistics), the TCP/IP (Transmission Control Protocol / Internet Protocol) protocol stack and the devices or wireless accesses. The CCF is built around three main principles that guarantee a simple and flexible architecture, which could be summed up in a modification of the terminal operating system.

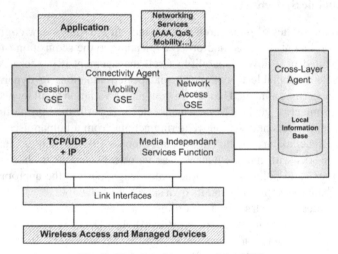

Fig. 2. Global architecture of the CCF

The main principle is to hide the heterogeneity and diversity of the devices and access networks behind an abstract interface which facilitates a range of services wider than handover management. This is achieved by the Media Independent Services Function (MISF) and the Link Interfaces. Another principle is to share the knowledge about the terminal context and its environment between the different components in a cross-layer fashion. This is achieved by the Cross-Layer Agent (CLA) which stores the configuration, policies and statuses in a Local Information Base (LIB). Finally, generic service enablers (GSEs), integrated in a Connectivity

Agent (CA) take care of dedicated basic service operations. They enhance the terminal operational behaviour for an autonomous and optimized connectivity, coping with dynamic changes and events in its environment.

3.2 MIS Functions and Managed Interfaces

The MISF is an abstraction layer which deals with the wireless multimodality of the terminal. It is a key component of the system, as it provides the means for the abstracted interaction between the wireless accesses or other devices and the upper layers, hiding their individual specificities. It is based on the MIH services, but is not restricted to handover. It provides a whole set of additional services, including monitoring of access networks, retrieving of system statistics and status, resource configuration with a certain level of Quality of Service (QoS), handling power sources, positioning device or enabling multicast and broadcast services.

At the lower layer, the Link Interfaces make the link between the MISF and the technologies device drivers. There is one Link Interface per type of device, completely specific to its implementation. Its main function is to translate the MIS commands and forward them downwards to the target driver. It acts as the endpoint for parameters retrieval in the upwards direction, possibly scheduling some periodic monitoring of the device. It receives the configuration MIS primitives and executes internal procedures to enable the reporting of measurements or subscribed events. Its location at the edge of the CCF minimizes the overall energy and processing power consumed by the framework. The Link Interfaces for the wireless devices control the access technologies present in the terminal. Nevertheless, a mobile terminal, whether it is a laptop, smartphone or OBU, includes devices other than the wireless interfaces, e.g. positioning systems, power supplies or tags and light sensors. In the same manner as the wireless interfaces, these devices can be controlled and monitored. When they relate to the mobile connectivity, they enhance its coordinated and integrated control through the CCF and the MISF, provided the availability of a specific Link Interface. Using this feature may prove very interesting as the OBU would be able to retrieve the speed of the car to eliminate the cells with small coverage, e.g., WLAN (Wireless Local Area Network) from the access selection decision.

A simplified set of primitives can be defined to make the MIS interactions generic. A Link_Action primitive carries a command from the upper layers. In the reverse direction, the Link_Report indicates an information from the Link Interface. The Link_Information is used by the MISF to exchange parameter values with the LIB, while the Link_Configure registers subscriptions for specific measurement reports from the device through the Link Interface. With these procedures, the MISF and the Link Interfaces bring to the framework the capability to manage, in an abstracted and flexible way, the various network interfaces and devices present in a terminal in order to achieve an optimized connectivity.

3.3 Network Access Selection

In the CA, the Network Access Generic Service Enabler (NAGSE) deals with aspects related to the monitoring of the networks availability, learning the characteristics of the unknown accesses and selecting the best network by running its algorithm on a set of parameters retrieved from the CLA. For the discovery and monitoring of available networks, it uses mainly the information received by the network interfaces, either to identify the availability of a known network or to learn the system information from an unknown network: radio technology, network name, signal quality, capabilities and available bandwidth.

The access network selection algorithm in the NAGSE may be invoked by the autonomous coordination function in the CA from several different states of the system. When the terminal starts, it is called to identify the initial network to attach to, without any running application. When a new application starts, it is requested to check whether the connected network is suitable. If several are available at once (in case of multi-homing for example), it evaluates which one is the most convenient. The objective is to apply an algorithm to a set of parameters and derive a configuration, in the form of the preferred ordered list of access networks, according to known policies. The criteria introduced by the policies govern the following metrics: better coverage, connectivity stability, load balancing, energy efficiency, application requirements in terms of bandwidth, QoS, technology or network support, capacity stability and network security. The most widely used algorithm, the SAW, is chosen here to compute the decision, because it is simple, converges in a limited amount of time and requires a reduced processing time since only one score value per access network has to be calculated. The score S_i of the current context for the i-th target network is determined thanks to a single calculation as

$$S_i = \sum_{j=1}^{n} w_j.r_{ij}$$

where w_j is the link reward of parameter j for the target application and the access network considered and r_{ij} is the measured value of the j-th parameter of the i-th network. The different scores allow to determine an ordered list of (access network, score) pairs. Because the algorithm depends on a combination of a discrete number of parameters and link rewards in a limited number of cases, it converges very rapidly. It allows using a larger set of attributes and thus reflects more closely the userand terminal context. Moreover, this algorithm is very flexible. It is easier to add a parameter than with "if then else" policies because it only requires that the new attribute get allocated link reward values. These values are determined by the CLA which is the component responsible of the learning process in the CCF. Based on the feedback from the user and the physical environment received through the other components, it analyses the values of parameters and policies that have been applied to determine the rewards that can optimize the operation of the CCF. With these functionalities, the NAGSE brings to the framework the capability to characterize the network environment in a very precise manner and to select the best access network for each application, taking into account several independent criteria in a flexible algorithm. The coordination of the MISF abstract interface with the NAGSE allows the system to operate in an autonomous and more dynamic manner.

4   Validating the Framework

To enable the evaluation of the benefits of the CCF operation, a prototype has been developed, using the OMNET++ platform [10], a discrete event simulation system. The simulation executes Ping connection tests or a web browsing application in a mobile terminal which moves randomly across a heterogeneous network playground, while the rest of the system parameters remain unchanged. This choice of applications allows demonstrating the dynamicity and efficiency of the framework. Figure 3 shows the network layout used for the simulation.

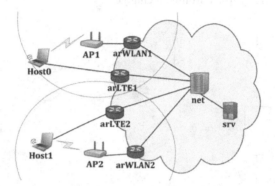

Fig. 3. Simulated network scenario

The LTE cell has a global coverage and provides an always-on access, while the WLAN availability is restricted to the circle shown in the picture around each access point. The results of the CCF prototype development are compared with two other cases: single technology (stationary WLAN) wireless terminal and mobile terminal equipped with a CMGR which fosters the WLAN access, in order to get the largest bandwidth and reduce the communication cost. The CCF module implemented strictly follows the architecture described in Section 3. Fifty simulation runs with random MT movements are executed for each test case in order to obtain a better confidence in the set of results. The main success criterion is the minimization of the number of broken sessions and packets lost, showing that the MTs obtained a suited connectivity at every position of the playground. The following metrics are collected: number of bytes transmitted and received by the applications, number of TCP connections opened / broken during the test, number of Echo Request packets sent and Echo Reply packets received back during the Ping test.

The results obtained are shown in Figure 4. Figure 4a pictures the measurements obtained with the Ping test. With the stationary WLAN, the terminal remains under the coverage of the wireless cell for the whole simulation, so no packet is lost. When the terminal moves and the CMGR switches the connectivity, between 3 and 7 packets, with an average of 3 packets, are lost for the time of the simulation. When the CCF replaces the CMGR, the loss rate drops to 0%, similar to the stationary WLAN use case. This result is due to the capability brought by the MISF to early report a vanishing network, and thus enable the upper layers to transfer immediately the connectivity to another available link before the older one is broken. Figure 4b shows the number of broken sessions (–BRK) according to the total number of opened sessions (–ALL) for the interactive web browsing application. With the stationary WLAN, 400 sessions are successfully started; the number of broken sessions is equal to zero. With the CMGR, fewer sessions can be established and several sessions are broken while they are executing. When using the CCF, the number of broken session is reduced to zero. All the sessions are successful. A very small amount of requests are retried by the application because the downlink packets were lost during the network change. These results confirm that the CCF terminal could adapt successfully to environment changes.

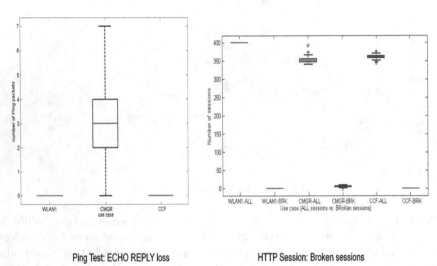

Ping Test: ECHO REPLY loss   HTTP Session: Broken sessions

Fig. 4. Comparison of simulation results when using the CCF

In order to evaluate the impact of the CCF on the terminal processing time, a sample typical test has been made to measure the amount of discrete events involving the CCF and Link Interfaces components, vs. the total number of events for the whole simulation run. Table 1 shows the measured values for a specific test session. The additional number of discrete events introduced by the CCF remains under 0.2% of the total number of events.

Table 1. Measured processing time

	Number of events executed	**Percentage**
Total of the simulation	761839	
ccf contribution	409	0.0537%
Link Interfaces contribution	824	0.1082%

Another validation activity has consisted in applying the concept of abstraction from the technology specificities to real sub-systems, as described below.

In the first use case, the MIS have been implemented to support QoS resource allocation together with seamless mobility, targeting the integration in a beyond-3G cellular access. In this system, the upper layers were directly the Mobility management and the QoS controller and enforcement entities, showcasing the flexibility of the MISF abstraction. The performance parameters taken into account were the average delay, the packet loss and the jitter. During the tests, the average handover delay has been measured at around 6 seconds, with a non-significant disruption time. This result was expected because the new network attachment is performed before the old one is broken. For the same reason, it was confirmed that the packet loss was null during the handovers. Finally, the jitter measured at the MT during each handover was at the same level as the jitter obtained in a stable situation.

The second use case has addressed the Management layer of the OBU, a vertical cross-layer component, where the communication technology selection decides of the most suitable set of communication protocols and access technologies to carry the messages of a given ITS application. A specificity of ITS communications is that this decision must be made according to the type of the message or flow to transmit. It is closely related with the application which indicates its own requirements and the current context of the device. The global process is pictured in Figure 5.

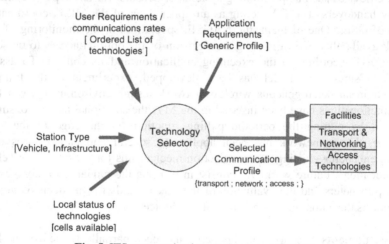

Fig. 5. ITS communications technology selection

The first input consists in the type of the originating and destination terminal. It may be a vehicle, a RSU (Road Side Unit) or a central traffic station. The second set of inputs is user-originated. Based on user preferences and subscription rates, the Management layer builds dynamically an ordered list of access networks. In the case of a central station, this list is built by matching the destination target area geography with the topology of transmitting stations (base stations or RSUs) covering that area. The process receives from the application the profile requirement associated to the message type. The same type of message (e.g., event notification) may have different values under different conditions or applications. The fourth and last input is built from the station context and contains the current status of the network accesses, observed locally, with parameters such as signal quality, radio coverage, network load or distance to the destination terminal. The objective of the decision is to choose the most suitable communication profile which includes the Transport protocol, the Network protocol and the Access technology.

This approach has been applied to the implementation of the communication technology selector in a simulation platform and has led to the definition of two procedures, the first one applied to the vehicle decision process and a second one applied to the global infrastructure (central station) decision process. They have provided very successful results.

5   Conclusion

A cross-layer and integrated framework for handling autonomously heterogeneous interfaces, the Connectivity Control Framework, has been proposed in this paper. The approach adopted here is that the CCF is restricted to the MT and has no impact on the mobile network infrastructure. It includes an abstraction layer which hides the network specificities to the rest of the framework and includes the support of other hardware devices such as positioning systems or sensors, for any type of control and not only handovers. The CA, acting as an upper layer of the MISF, coordinates the actions of GSEs. One of them, the NAGSE, specializes in the monitoring of access network availability and in making the decision of the optimal access to be selected by the OBU according to the executing application and its context. To assess its benefits, a simulation model has been developed, experimenting the framework behaviour in an heterogeneous wireless network testing environment. Even though these functionalities have been inserted in the MT, the additional power consumption is limited by putting the periodic polling functions at the edge of the system. Moreover, this framework has been applied to several application cases on real systems, enhancing existing access selection mechanisms for the upcoming vehicular communications. Future work will consist in refining the modality of storage for the context parameters and the evaluation of the link rewards for the decision algorithm that supports the autonomous operation of the device.

Acknowledgments. The work in this paper has been partially funded fy the French DGCIS project SCORE@F (http://www.scoref.fr/)

References

1. European ITS Communication Architecture Overall Framework, COMeSafety project: http://www.comesafety.org
2. Piri, E., Pentikousis, K.: IEEE 802.21. The Internet Protocol Journal 12(2) (June 2009)

3. Yan, X., Ahmet Şekercioğlu, Y., Narayanan, S.: A survey of vertical handover decision algorithms in Fourth Generation heterogeneous wireless networks. Computer Networks 54(11) (August 2010)
4. Ahmad, S., Rohling, H. (dir.), Yin, C.: Multi-standard Convergence in Mobile Terminals (Master Thesis). Hamburg University of Technology (February 2005)
5. Corici, M., Diez, A., Vingarzan, D., Magedanz, T., Pampu, C., Qing, Z.: Enhanced access network discovery and selection in 3GPP Evolved Packet Core. In: IEEE 34th Conference on Local Computer Networks, Zurich, October 20-23 (2009)
6. Kassar, M., Kervella, B., Pujolle, G.: An overview of vertical handover decision strategies in heterogeneous wireless networks. Computer Communications 31(10) (June 2008)
7. Stevens-Navarro, E., Lin, Y., Wong, V.W.S.: An MDP-Based Vertical Handoff Decision Algorithm for Heterogeneous Wireless Networks. IEEE Transactions on Vehicular Technology 57(2) (March 2008)
8. Larsen, J.: Cognitive Systems. Tutorial presented at IEEE Workshop on Machine Learning for Signal Processing, Cancun, Mexico (October 2008)
9. IBM Corporation: An Architectural Blueprint for Autonomic Computing. White Paper, 4th edn. (June 2006)
10. http://www.omnetpp.org/

A 3.4-GHz Double Patch Pike-Shape Antenna for Wireless Applications

Constantinos T. Angelis[*], Eirini Tsiakalou, and Christos Koliopanos

Department of Informatics and Telecommunications,
Technological Educational Institute of Epirus, Arta, Greece
kangelis@teiep.gr, {etsiak,xkoliopanos}@teleinfom.teiep.gr

Abstract. The goal of this paper is to investigate the performance of double patch printed antenna for wireless applications. The antenna is characterized in terms of impedance bandwidth, gain and radiation patterns through simulations. Simulations present satisfactory radiation pattern. The proposed antenna has the advantage of compact size, which makes it attractive for mobile devices.

Index Terms: Ultra-Wideband, Printed antennas, WiMax.

1   Introduction

During the last years there has been tremendous growth in wireless communication technology, especially for the IEEE 802.16 and IEEE 802.20 Worldwide Interoperability for Microwave Access (WiMAX) standards. Many researchers work in designing single, dual and tri-band antennas for WLAN/WiMAX applications [1-7]. The proposed antenna has the advantage of compact size, which makes it attractive for mobile devices.

The remaining of this paper is organized as follows: Section 2 describes the basic antenna design; Section 3 presents the simulation results and extensive numerical and simulation evidence of the proposed antenna; and the conclusions are given in Section 4.

2   Antenna Design

The proposed antenna is etched on a substrate of thickness 1.52 mm and dielectric constant of 3.38. The substrate has a compact dimension of 30 x 40mm^2. Fig. 2 shows the structure of the proposed antenna. The antenna consists of a single layer, which is the radiating layer as the ground plane of the antenna is located on the same side of the CPW-feed and radiating portion. The antenna is simulated using the parameters given in Table 1. The complete 3D structure is presented in Fig. 2 where it is possible to observe the patch of the antenna and its feeding plate.

Fig. 1 shows a pike-shape patch that is excited by a microstrip line through EM coupling.

---

[*] Member IEEE, ICST, EuMA.

C.T. Angelis, D. Fotiadis, and A.T. Tzallas (Eds.): AMBI-SYS 2013, LNICST 118, pp. 104–112, 2013.

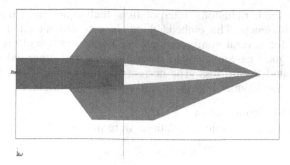

Fig. 1. Two dimensional structure of the proposed pike-shape double patch antenna

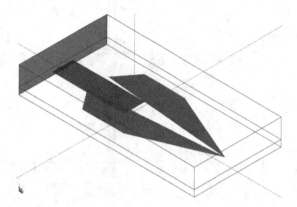

Fig. 2. Three dimensional structure of the proposed pike-shape double patch antenna

3   Results and Discussion

To verify our design approach and in parallel the effectiveness and feasibility of the proposed design we used simulation with ADS software. Simulations performed with Method of Moments and Finite Element Method. The Method of Moments was used to find the resonant frequency of the proposed antenna.   A moment method analysis of planar circuits in a layered medium is developed. The Green's functions of a two-layer grounded medium are used in order to take into account the effect of the surface

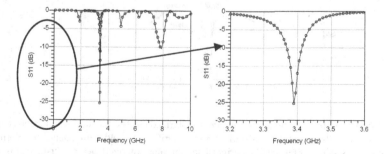

Fig. 3. Simulated reflection coefficient versus frequency

wave, coupling, and radiation. Interpolation techniques are used to increase computational efficiency. The embedded conductors are modeled with triangular patches. Results for several configurations, including direct and proximity coupled radiators, are in good agreement with measurements and other calculations. Fig. 3 shows the simulated Return loss. The current is predominantly excited at the pike-shape patch. The Bandwidth of the proposed antenna is 250MHz.

A. 2-D Far Field Calculations at 3.4 GHz

Two dimensional (2-D) far field calculations were performed with the Finite Element Method.

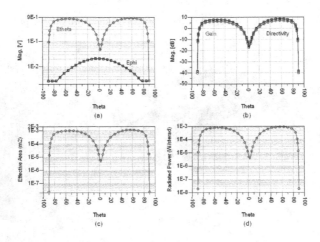

Fig. 4. (a) Absolute field strength (in volts) of the theta and phi electric far-field components, (b) Gain, Directivity, (c) Effective area (in m2), (d) Radiation intensity (in Watts/steradian), in the XZ-plane

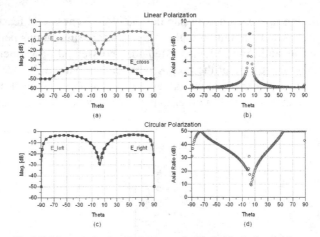

Fig. 5. (a) Normalized field strength of co and cross polarized electric far-field components, (b) Axial ratio, derived from left-hand and right-hand circular polarized far-field components, (c) Normalized field strength of respectively left-hand and right-hand circular polarized electric far-field component, (d) Linear polarization axial ratio, derived from co and cross polarized far-field components

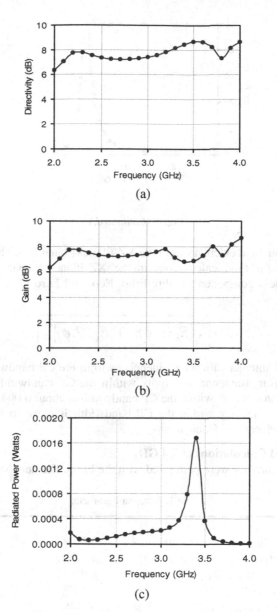

Fig. 6. (a) Directivity, (b) Gain, (c) Radiated Power and (d) % Injected Power versus frequency

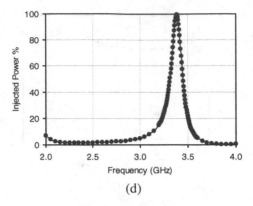

(d)

Fig. 6. (*Continued.*)

Fig. 5 shows far field calculations in the XZ-Plane (Planar Cut, phi=0).

Fig. 6 shows far field calculations in the XZ-Plane (Planar Cut, phi=0). The normalized far-field components (Elhp, Erhp, Eco, and Ecross) are normalized with respect to:

$$
\max\left(\sqrt{\left|E_\theta(\theta,\phi)\right|^2 + \left|E_\phi(\theta,\phi)\right|^2} \right).
$$

The measured antenna gain for frequencies within the CP bandwidth is about 6.8–7.8 dBi, the measured antenna directivity within the CP bandwidth is about 7.8–8.4 dBi and the Radiated Power within the CP bandwidth is about 0.004 to 0.0018 Watts.

The radiation efficiency within the CP bandwidth is close to 80%, and remains constant in both Planar and Conical cuts.

B. 3-D Far Field Calculations at 3.4 GHz
3-D far field calculations were performed with the Finite Element Method.

Table 1. Antenna Parameters

Resonant Frequency (GHz)	3.4	
Radiated power (Watts)	0.00167	
Effective angle (Steradians)	1.78818	
Directivity (dB)	8.46798	
Gain (dB)	6.80792	
Maximum radiation intensity (Watts/Steradian)	0.00094	
Direction of maximum radiation intensity (theta, phi), (degrees)	57	0
E(theta) max (magnitude, phase)	0.83996	-134.7
E(phi) max (magnitude, phase)	0.00664	25.5
E(x) max (magnitude, phase)	0.45748	-134.7
E(y) max (magnitude, phase)	0.00664	25.5
E(z) max (magnitude, phase)	0.70445	45.3

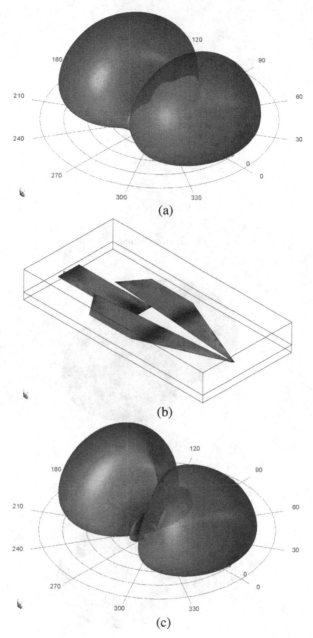

Fig. 7. (a) 3-D Normalized E, (b) Animation snapshot of the electric field in all directions, (c) Normalized ETheta and (d) Normalized EPhi, for the 3.4 GHz

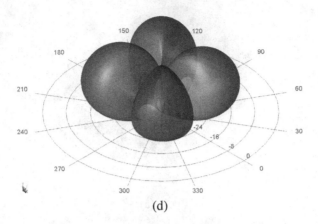

(d)

Fig. 7. (*Continued.*)

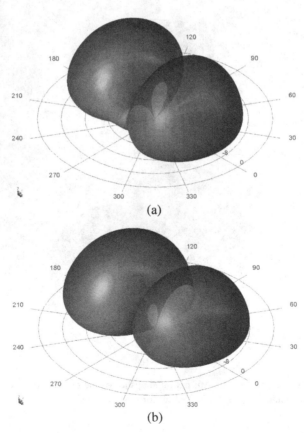

(a)

(b)

Fig. 8. 3-D Normalized (**a**) ELeft, (**b**) ERight (**c**) ECo and (**d**) ECross, for the 3.4 GHz

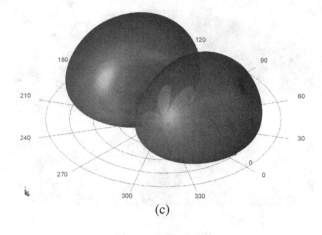

(c)

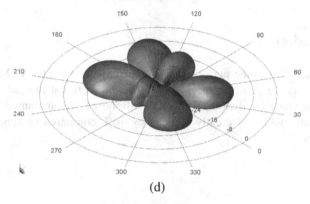

(d)

Fig. 8. (*Continued.*)

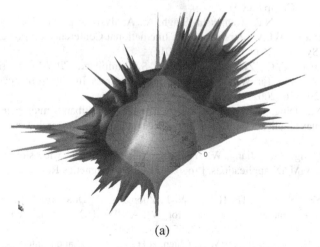

(a)

Fig. 9. 3-D Normalized (**a**) Linear Axial Ratio, (**b**) Circular Axial Ratio, for the 3.4 GHz

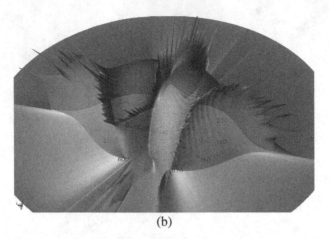

(b)

Fig. 9. (*Continued.*)

4   Conclusion

In this paper we focus on the performance of a printed antenna for WiMax (3.4 GHz) applications. It has the good characteristics of omnidirectional radiation patterns and very wide impedance bandwidth. The total volume of the antenna is 20 (L)x7.64 (W)x0.4 (H) mm^3, which is greatly reduced by 36% compared to generally internal printed radiators.

References

[1] Batra, A.: MultiBand OFDM physical layer specification. MultiBand OFDM Alliance Special Interest Group (2005)

[2] Mishra, A., Yadav, N.P., Kamakshi, Singh, A.: Analysis of pair of L-shaped slot loaded patch antenna for WLAN application. In: International Conference on Power, Control and Embedded Systems (ICPCES), pp. 1–5 (2010)

[3] Song, Y., Jiao, Y.-C., Zhao, G., Zhang, F.-S.: Multiband CPW-FED Triangle-Shaped Monopole Antenna for Wireless Applications. Progress In Electromagnetics Research, PIER 70, 329–336 (2007)

[4] Song, Z.-N., Ding, Y., Huang, K.: A compact multiband monopole antenna for WLAN/wimax applications. Progress In Electromagnetics Research Letters 23, 147–155 (2011)

[5] Zhao, Q., Gong, S.-X., Jiang, W., Yang, B., Xie, J.: Compact wide-slot tri-band antenna for WLAN/WiMAX applications. Progress In Electromagnetics Research Letters 18, 9–18 (2010)

[6] Kang, L., Yin, Y.-Z., Li, H., Huang, W.-J., Zheng, S.-F.: Dual-wideband symmetrical G-shaped slotted monopole antenna for WLAN/WiMAX applications. Progress In Electromagnetics Research Letters 17, 55–65 (2010)

[7] Chien, Y.P., Horng, T.S., Chen, W.S., Chien, H.H.: Dual wideband printed monopole antenna for WLAN/WiMAX applications. IEEE Antennas Wireless Propag. Lett. 6, 149–151 (2007)

Mobile Widget Technology as a Solution for Smart User Interaction

Miroslav Behan and Ondrej Krejcar

University of Hradec Kralove, FIM, Department of Information Technologies,
Rokitanskeho 62,Hradec Kralove, 500 03, Czech Republic
Miroslav.Behan@uhk.cz, Ondrej.Krejcar@remoteworld.net

Abstract. Widget technology will increase its potential in time due to visualization comprehensiveness, fast content reachability and easy event driven possibilities. The most positive factor of spreading widget technology world widely is usability for tasks on daily bases. Widget users are not bordered pointless middle steps to acquired correct information. The widget technology will shape modern view of applicant use due to utilization software platforms leads by simultaneously of mobile devices increasing influence. We would see future in user friendly environment where are interactions with surroundings devices based on simple, smart and customizable widgets, gadgets or plugins.

Keywords: Widget, Mobile, Device, User, Interaction, GUI.

1 Introduction

The access to content is nowadays driven mainly by web or mobile application bases and therefore the changing of human behavior in cyberspace shaped by mobile devices is recognized as an increasing influence of application design where intuitivism and user experience are on the first place. The mobile applications, which conceptually are enhanced with easy, fast and understandable content bundled into simple application package consists of graphics, code and in some cases external resources, is due to necessity of small and handy mobile device resolutions perfect environment which impacts development for higher user experience. Also that pushes development design level further to designing applications with real importance according to content delivery and applicability. Other motivation which speeds up application evolution process is covered in user's feedback possibility and is called market place environment where applications are rated by users according to satisfaction of goals and quality of user experiences. And also identification of mobile applications which are expressed by visualized icon and simple words benefits over current main domain name of identification for web application. The informational stream or content could be directly accessed by single user touch thought widgets technology and there is no need to remember or type correct domain name and load whole web content repeatedly to get daily bases kind of information but just simple to have a look on home screen where all required content is already loaded with actual information.

C.T. Angelis, D. Fotiadis, and A.T. Tzallas (Eds.): AMBI-SYS 2013, LNICST 118, pp. 113–122, 2013.
© Institute for Computer Sciences, Social Informatics and Telecommunications Engineering 2013

2   Problem Definition of Widget Technology

The fast, intuitive and easy to use access for basic devices features by widget technology is an issue over the specific platforms. The concept of widget technology comes historically from desktop computers where users could extract fragments of functionality or information of desktop to defined area. The usability of such kind of content is positive and could be also negative in specific cases. The inconvenient behavior could be caused by incorrect design or fragmented aim of informational stream in terms of remote based information provided by 3rd part provider. We describe in this chapter history of technology, platforms overview and architectural aspects. Typical widget became common on desktop computers where the story of 3rd side reusable small applications starts. We could call them also gadgets, portlets, modules or plugins and we could divide them by background used technologies or by type of client. At first types are simple categorized into desktop, web, mobile or TV widgets. For further more granulation let's focus on technological point of view which are used and are typical for widgets. In case of web background we recognized types as HTML + JavaScript, Adobe Flash, SilverLight or Java applet. These widgets could be embedded in website as well as ported into desktop widgets by particular container as Webkit, Adobe AIR, SilverLight Desktop or Java Virtual Machine. This kind of solution is preferred in case of high needs of variability and portability but could not equally supplement native desktop client application due to specific system functions restrictions. Therefore the desktop widgets are better solutions in case of more system or hardware functionality requirements for instance as hardware

Table 1. Mobile Platform Comparison [1]

Platform	Android	iOS	Windows Phone 7
Developer	Google	Apple	Microsoft
Copy/Paste	Yes	Yes	-
Multitasking	Yes	Yes	-
Flash Support	Yes	-	-
SilverLight Support	-	-	-
HTML5 Support	Yes	Yes	-
Unified Inbox	Yes	Yes	-
Exchange Support	Yes	Yes	Yes
Threaded Email	Yes	Yes	-
Visual Voicemail	Yes	Yes	-
Video Calling	Yes (3rd side)	Yes	-
Universal Search	Yes	Yes	-
Internet Tethering	Yes	Yes	-
Removable Storage	Yes	-	-
Folders	Yes	Yes	Hubs
Widgets Technology	Yes	-	Tiles on Home Screen

monitoring or operational system calls which are not implemented in containers for web widgets because of multiple platforms consistency. The desktop widgets are developed mostly as clones of C objective language such as C# (Windows), C++ (Unix) or Object-C (Mac OS) and also with popular Java (any JVM embedded). Others alternatives are developed in Perl (Unix) or Visual Basic (Windows) dependable on desired platform of use. Mobile widgets are nowadays fast growing area which is fully supported on Android. Others mobile platforms partial or even not support widget technology at all (see fig.1).

The next chapters we will focus on descriptions problematic cross platforms and at last we mentions future heading of TV widgets.

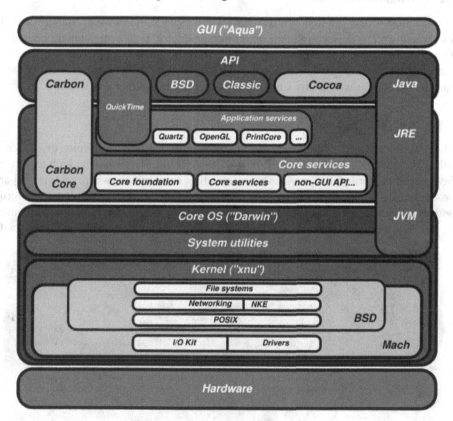

Fig. 1. Apple OS X Architecture [2]

2.1   Apple Platform

The solution based on Apple platform provides for developers fundamental and well prepared design support with framework named COCOA, which is basically using Object-C as programmatic language. There are others extensions from point of developers view where Java or others scripting languages could be used and also when we talked about apple platform we have to announce there are two operation systems the iOS for mobile devices and OS X (see fig.1) for desktops. The differences are in architectural aspects and supportive environmental tools. Undependable on system bases the most convenient way for developing application or widget applications are in usage common system calls as application interfaces, application services and core services (see figure 1). The advantage of apple platform is basically comprehensive, publishable and distributive widget channel over internet by widgets download center but only for desktop applications. Mobile devices widgets are not supported and therefore the usability of iOS is by this inconvenience decreased.

2.2   Windows Platform

The desktop widget applications are known for users Windows XP, Windows Vista and Windows 7 as desktop gadgets used through sidebar as docking content container. The comprehensive user's environment and easy installation process represent high usability of 3rd side content providing. However Windows Phone is only provide partial solution for widgets by simple tiles which trigger widget application.

2.3   Android Platform

The mobile platform which enables full widget technology and suits to designed solution which is described in next chapter is Android platform. The architecture of Java based platform fully provides multithreading environment where widgets [6] are processed by application widget provider which for defined scheduled time rerun widget application process for limited amount of time where over time consummation is not allowed and the process is killed. The widget would be designed with

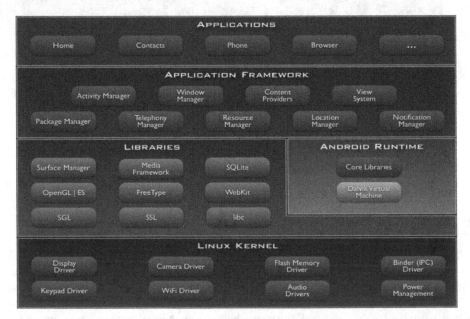

Fig. 2. Android Architecture [3]

responsible battery management and processing time. In case of usage more complicated tasks as internet resource or web services gathering there are allowed services which are running on background and the widget process itself could be only as initializer of background service. The visualization of widgets is based on RemoteViews classes which defines views for particular content and are representation also of user interface in terms of events triggering. For better overview following figure represents Android architecture (see figure 2).

2.4   TV Platform

Last band new area of widgets usage is television platforms where directions we evolution we recognized more in change of TV rather than TV embedded solution. For instance some of vendors supports embedded widget engine based on XML+JS for instance Konfabulator but with low reflection in mass use and there for others vendors as Samsung who directly comes with whole embedded platform Android in TV called Smart TV would change establishment and reality of understanding what television really is.

3   Solution Design

This chapter overviewed application development solution which is based on widget technology and provides core mobile devices functionality. In term of usability we decided to develop such widget application where user could easily control mobile devices features with simple one click functionality. The concept and implementation is based on Android and programed in Java with well-known application architecture model view control (MVC) concept. As visualization of views is used customized component which change its status dependable on mobile device features status change or by user's required actions (see figure 3). Model component represents feature's functionality and provides access to system call or platform API which are allowed. Control component of concept receiving and sending broadcast event and control behavior of view and model component. View in terms of MVC concept we called as a

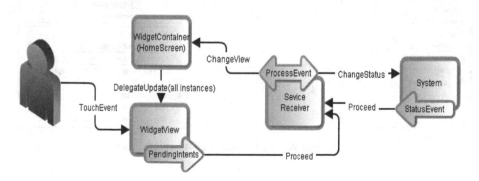

Fig. 3. Mobile Widget Architecture - Events

layout which consist of widgets or other layouts and views based on XML configuration file. In eclipse android plug-in there is a standard palette of views, layouts and widgets. Also developers could define their own views where it is overwritten by *onDraw()* method of *View* class. All raster graphical resources have to be assigned in *res* folder of project specified by type of resolution for concrete device screen.

The essential for application architecture as widgets is message driven model which responses on customized service calls which leads to widget view update. All services are in consideration of one service pattern which interacts with system. The views are managed by widget container which also handles user events called *PendingIntent.* The user events are posted to correct receiver and invoke inner process as an application owner. Process called as Service or Receiver is responsible for view updates and interaction with system. For better overview we outlined following class diagram (see figure 4) and describe application in more detail.

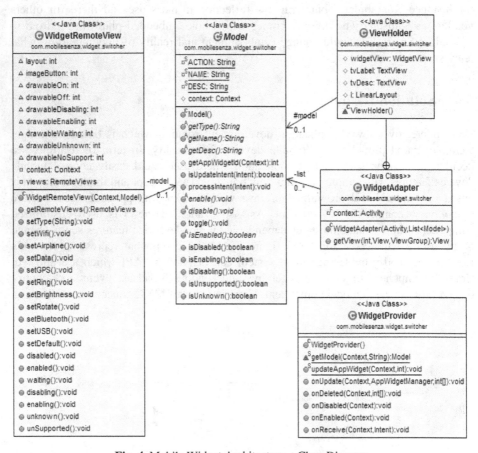

Fig. 4. Mobile Widget Architecture – Class Diagram

The *WidgetRemoteView* class is responsible for correct visualization and user event handling of all widgets. Basically is a container for customized view in easy and comprehensive way of approach to *RemoteViews* class which in terms of Android architecture is fundamental for widget concept. All widget instances are maintained by widget manager and therefore Views of widgets are not directly accessible therefore the only consistent way of changing widget views or associated user actions is by delegating *RemoteViews* instances to widget manager. For communication with widget manager is responsible *WidgetProvider* class which generating correspondent *RemoteViews* by method *getRemoteViews()* and post them by *updateAppWidget()*. The user's actions are represented by *PendingIntent* class as an event which could trigger 3rd side *Service* or *Receiver* due to consistency of developed authorization mechanism. The access is encoded by definition of Intent and we could consider them as authorization tokens with message based delivery which triggers particular task. The Model abstract class is pattern for all device features model classes which could be handled by known states as a enable, disable, toggle methods are connected to system calls and changing the statuses of desired feature accordingly to user defined service permissions. Finally *WidgetAdapter* class represents list container for all implemented modeled features of device to overview statuses on one place in real-time [9], [13] and also as choice optionality for widget selection before placement on home screen [5].

4   Testing Use Case Application – Widget Switcher

The *Widget Switch* is mobile application enables, disables or change status of specific mobile device features. The application is available on Google Play market for any device with Android [4]. We implement following (see table 1) mobile device features based on toggle buttons which are displaying status and are for touch screen events responsible to correspondent system change. Core application is running in background service which is driven by widgets. The widgets are places over widget native device selector on any place on home screens. All instances of the same type of toggle widget are changing upon system status change at the same time.

Widget switch is free for download application where we consider many possible extensions as other device features to be widget like controlled as a system monitoring tools (processor, networks, and memory), external service informational content providing, environment context status resolver, cost/effective communication connectivity, financial data overviewing, etc. We outline just subset possibilities of huge range of widget technology usage.

Table 2. Implemented Android Features Overview

Widget	States	Description
Wifi-WLAN	Disabled Enabling Enabled Disabling Unknown	The functionality is based upon system calls or receives of WLAN radio status. The connectivity to concrete wireless network is beyond application based on configuration and network priority policy [7], [8]
Air Mode	On Off	Mode of in airplane device behavior where could be specified also omitted or included networks explicitly.
Bluetooth	Disabled Enabling Enabled Disabling Unknown	The Bluetooth radio is behave on android platform close to wireless radio where widget application only enables or disables Bluetooth connectivity.
Brightness	Auto Manual	Settings auto is corresponding with saving battery policy; manual values are in 0-100% interval.
GPS	Enable Disable	From 2.3 Android version is only navigate over link to native settings.
Ring	On Silent Vibrate	Status of incoming calls where on is defined ring tone, vibrate only or silent for mute all.

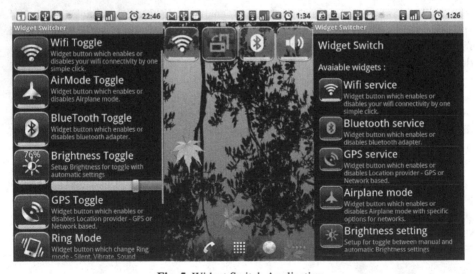

Fig. 5. Widget Switch Application

5   Conclusions

The widget based technology empowers usability of corresponding platform whether is desktop or mobile device. Widgets would be ideal extensions for common applications where summarized data or fast user reaction is required. The advantages of widget technology will be revealed with emerging mobile device and television widget platforms market where 3rd side content providers are required by advantages of mass creative content human power. Presented solution is also usable in numerous cases of image or video processing solutions [10-19], where it can significantly speed up usage by intuitive design.

Acknowledgement. This work was supported partially by (1) "Smart Solutions in Ubiquitous Computing Network Environments", Grant Agency of Excellence, University of Hradec Kralove, Faculty of Informatics and Management under the project GAE/2012/2213 and (2) "SmartHomePoint Solutions for Ubiquitous Computing Environments", University of Hradec Kralove under the project SP/2013.

References

1. PCWorld mobile platform comparisation, http://www.pcworld.com/article/208491/mobile_os_smackdown_windows_phone_7_vs_ios_vs_android.html (retrieved October 22, 2010)
2. Apple Developer Site, iOS, https://developer.apple.com/library/ios/#documentation/ (retrieved May 24, 2012)
3. Wikipedia, Android OS, http://en.wikipedia.org/wiki/Android_(operating_system) (retrieved May 23, 2012)
4. Widget Switch Application, Google Play Marketplace, https://play.google.com/store/apps/details?id=com.mobilesenza.widget.switcher
5. Komatineni, S., MacLean, D., Hashimi, S.Y.: Home Screen Widgets, Pro Android 3, pp. 711–743 (2011), doi:10.1007/978-1-4302-3223-0_22
6. Murphy, M.L.: Beginning Android 2, Employing Fancy Widgets and Containers, pp. 95–116 (2010), doi:10.1007/978-1-4302-2630-7_9
7. Machaj, J., Brida, P.: Impact of Radio Fingerprints Processing on Localization Accuracy of Fingerprinting Algorithms. Elektronika ir Elektrotechnika 18(7), 129–132 (2012), doi:10.5755/j01.eee.123.7.2391
8. Brida, P., Machaj, J., Gaborik, F., Majer, N.: Performance analysis of positioning in wireless sensor networks. Przeglad Elektrotechniczny 87(5), 257–260 (2011)
9. Herrero, A., Navarro, M., Corchado, E., Julian, V.: RT-MOVICAB-IDS: Addressing real-time intrusion detection. Future Generation Computer Systems 29(1), 250–261 (2013) ISSN 0167-739X, doi:10.1016/j.future.2010.12.017
10. Cheng, W.C., Liou, J.W., Liou, C.Y.: Construct Adaptive Template Array for Magnetic Resonance Images. In: IEEE International Joint Conference on Neural Networks, Brisbane, Australia, June 10-15 (2012), doi:10.1109/IJCNN.2012.6252560

11. Penhaker, M., Darebnikova, M., Cerny, M.: Sensor Network for Measurement and Analysis on Medical Devices Quality Control. In: Yonazi, J.J., Sedoyeka, E., Ariwa, E., El-Qawasmeh, E. (eds.) ICeND 2011. CCIS, vol. 171, pp. 182–196. Springer, Heidelberg (2011)
12. Machacek, Z., Slaby, R., Hercik, R., Koziorek, J.: Advanced System for Consumption Meters with Recognition of Video Camera Signal. Elektronika ir Elektrotechnika 18(10), 57–60 (2012), doi:10.5755/j01.eee.18.10.3062
13. Machacek, Z., Srovnal Jr., V.: Communication Network Model for Industrial Control. In: Proceedings of the 9th RoEduNet IEEE International Conference, Sibiu, Romania, June 24-26, pp. 293–298 (2010)
14. Juszczyszyn, K., Nguyen, N.T., Kolaczek, G., Grzech, A., Pieczynska, A., Katarzyniak, R.: Agent-based approach for distributed intrusion detection system design. In: Alexandrov, V.N., van Albada, G.D., Sloot, P.M.A., Dongarra, J. (eds.) ICCS 2006. LNCS, vol. 3993, pp. 224–231. Springer, Heidelberg (2006)
15. Vybiral, D., Augustynek, M., Penhaker, M.: Devices for Position Detection. Journal of Vibroengineering 13(3), 531–535 (2011)
16. Sojka, M., Pisa, P., Faggioli, D., Cucinotta, T., Checconi, F., Hanzalek, Z., Lipari, G.: Modular software architecture for flexible reservation mechanisms on heterogeneous resources. Journal of Systems Architecture 57(4), 366–382 (2011), doi:10.1016/j.sysarc.2011.02.005
17. Kasik, V., Penhaker, M., Novák, V., Bridzik, R., Krawiec, J.: User interactive biomedical data web services application. In: Yonazi, J.J., Sedoyeka, E., Ariwa, E., El-Qawasmeh, E. (eds.) ICeND 2011. CCIS, vol. 171, pp. 223–237. Springer, Heidelberg (2011)
18. Behan, M., Krejcar, O.: The Concept of the Remote Devices Content Management. Journal of Computer Networks and Communications 2012, Article ID 194284, 7 p. (2012), doi:10.1155/2012/194284
19. Vybiral, D., Augustynek, M., Penhaker, M.: Devices for position detection. Journal of Vibroengineering 13(3), 531–535 (2011)

Ambient Systems for the Environmental Monitoring: Characteristic Examples at Different Spatial Scales

Stavros Kolios[1] and Chrysostomos Stylios[2]

[1] Department of Applications of Information Technology in Administration and Economy,
TEI of Ionian Islands, 31100 Lefkada, Greece
stavroskolios@yahoo.gr

[2] Laboratory of Knowledge and Intelligent Computing (KIC-LAB), Department
of Informatics and Telecommunication Technology, TEI of Epirus, 47100, Arta, Greece
stylios@teiep.gr, stylios@teleinfom.teiep.gr

Abstract. This article is a short review highlighting the important role of ambient systems for the environmental monitoring. The article focuses on modern intelligent and fully automated systems that are able to use different kinds of data coming from scientific instrumentation and sensors as informational background in order to identify, analyze, monitor and forecast a vast series of parameters and phenomena that concern the atmosphere, the weather, land and seas. Here some characteristic examples of such systems are presented along with their basic operating principles, their usefulness and their perspectives in the environmental monitoring. Ambient systems have nowadays become essential solutions for the environmental monitoring and they are going to lead to the development of fully automated systems worldwide contributing in the efforts to preserve the Earth's environment.

Keywords: Ambient systems, environmental monitoring.

1   Introduction

Nowadays, the protection of the physical environment (land, ocean and atmosphere) is a major issue worldwide regarding the sustainable future and the improvement of quality of life. The role of computing and informatics is extremely important as can provide advanced automated systems. The recent advances at these two fields have led to modern, fully automated information systems able to handle, analyze, monitor and forecast (or model) a vast series of statiotemporal characteristics, parameters and phenomena that concern the atmosphere, the weather, land and seas.

Especially during the last decade new applications and systems have appeared providing solutions for analytic measuring, recording and monitoring of parameters and phenomena from local to large scale (Triantafyllou et al. [14], Chronis et al. [3] Kazantzidis et al. [7], Garcia-Sansez et al. [4], Hwang et al. [6]). Such systems belong to the "ambient systems" considering their general operational principles. Usually, they are based on networks of instruments/sensors (Fig. 1) and are deployed to improve environmental quality control, for example to monitor humidity and

C.T. Angelis, D. Fotiadis, and A.T. Tzallas (Eds.): AMBI-SYS 2013, LNICST 118, pp. 123–130, 2013.
© Institute for Computer Sciences, Social Informatics and Telecommunications Engineering 2013

temperatures in agricultural and other environments. Actually, the notion of ambient systems embeds the idea of large-scale heterogeneous systems being able to sense, network, inform, actuate and interact with the physical environment and the human. "These systems are at the heart of the next generation information technology, which will no longer be limited to dedicated infrastructures, such as the Internet, but will be embedded in artifacts and the environment and will consist of highly distributed, networked, heterogeneous, and largely self-organizing devices".

Ambient systems are developed and operated in different environmental applications accomplishing the special needs that are designed to serve, and providing by fully automated and intelligent way: data, products and solutions, by minimizing problems and diffusing information accurately and timely to the scientific community, governments, agencies, organizations and the citizens. Such systems provide environmental monitoring by measuring and analyzing environmental data over an unprecedented range of space and time scales using large-scale sensor networks, so that to accurately assess the impact of global warming, recognize and predict natural hazards (i.e. avalanches, floods, dangers, earthquakes, diseases), and support and manage sustainable land, water, and resource use. The general concept of ambient systems for environmental monitoring can be seen in fig. 1, differentiate according to the application but keeping the same, the general operating principles.

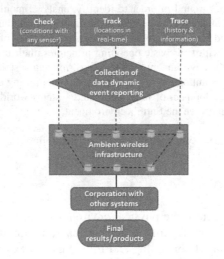

Fig. 1. General scheme of the ambient systems

2   Satellite Dissemination Systems

The most advanced, worldwide known and widely used ambient systems are the satellite data dissemination systems. Such systems have been operating for decades, they are continuously improved and expanding so that to cover the increasing needs of the scientific community. The sensors on board at the satellite platforms can collect all the appropriate information and automatically disseminate in real time basis on a network of ground stations. After all the necessary validation checking and the conversion on higher quality level data and products, all the users have access to such data and products in real time basis using their own ground station or as archived data from many dissemination facilities.

In Fig. 2 the dissemination system of Meteosat Second Generation (MSG) satellite data and products is presented as a characteristic example. The EUMETSAT (European Organization for the Exploitation of Meteorological Satellites) Application Ground Segment comprises a central processing facility and a distributed network of Satellite Application Facilities (SAF) that provide the necessary research, development, and generation of level 1 and level 2 satellite products for onward dissemination to the user community. The Central Application Facility (CAF) is responsible for the generation of level 1 processed satellite data and the generation of higher level 2 products, which primarily support the application needs for Nowcasting and Numerical Weather Prediction (NWP). The Satellite Application Facilities (SAFs) are a distributed network of thematic application facilities responsible for necessary research, development, and operational activities not carried out by the central facility.

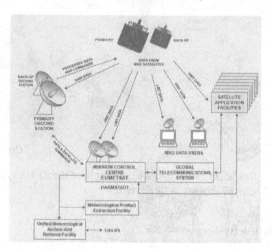

Fig. 2. A schematic data flow of Meteosat imagery from the satellite instruments to the user community network through validation, storage and product generation facilities

3   Large Scale Ambient Systems

There are two important sub categories of large scale environmental monitoring systems: the lightning detection systems and solar radiation systems.

3.1   Lightning Detection Systems

An interesting and important category of ambient systems is the networks of ground based sensors used to record lightning events during thunderstorms (e.g. "BrazilDAT", "LINET", "ZEUS", "ATD", "WWLLN"). The measurements of lightning events play a crucial role in the accurate detection of convection (e. g. Tadesse et al. [13], Mattos et al. [11]) and consequently they can provide valuable information to risk management and protection agencies. Such systems have increasingly developed and compared regarding their accuracy and their usefulness (e.g., Lagouvardos et al. [10], Kohn et al. [9])

A characteristic example of such systems is the Long Range Lightning Detection System with the code name "ZEUS" (Chronis et al. [3], Lagouvardos et al. [10]). The sensors of this network (Fig. 3b) can detect radio frequencies (sferics) released from lightning events at a range between 5 and 15 KHz (Chronis et al. [3]). The geographic location of every lightning event is calculated through a technique called "Arrival Time Difference Triangulation" and transmitted in real time basis to the central station of the network for further analysis, dissemination to the users and storage in the relative databases (Fig.3a).

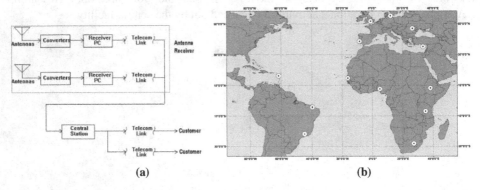

(a)   (b)

Fig. 3. a) A schematic flow chart of the operational stages of the ZEUS system, b) Geographic locations of the ZEUS sensors network at (green dots)

3.2   Solar Radiation Systems

The downwelling solar radiation is vital for every kind of life on Earth. Traditionally it is measured through scientific instrumentation at different locations. The spatial distribution of upwelling radiation can be measured accurately using sensors on board on the satellite platforms. But the downwelling radiation it can be measured. To alternate this restriction, especially during the last decade networks of instruments that measure downwelling radiance in many spectral regions has been developed so that to provide more information about the energy balance variations in the Earth's environment.

A characteristic example of such systems is called "UVNET". More analytically, since 2003, a Greek UV (UltraViolet) Network has been established and operated a number of stations in Greece and Cyprus (Fig. 4b). The instruments of the network are multichannel filter actinometers (Fig. 4a) and provide measurements of irradiance in the UV and the visible part of the solar spectrum. Other atmospheric parameters such total ozone, erythemal UV dose, cloud transmittance and photolysis rates can also be calculated using this network of sensors (Bais et al. [2], Kazantzidis et al. [7],

Kazantzidis et al. [8]). The final products of this system are presented in daily basis on the official website of the network (www.uvnet.gr).

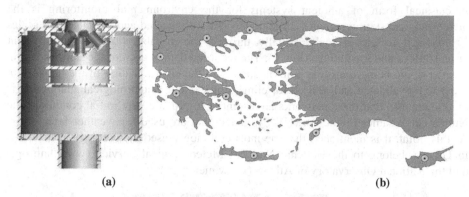

(a)   (b)

Fig. 4. a) Schematic representation of the actinometers used for measurements in the UV spectrum. b) The UV network (gray dots).

4   Micro Scale and Local Scale Ambient Systems

The most common ambient systems at micro or local scale for the environmental monitoring are those who are used in the agriculture sector. Indeed, it is well known that the monitoring of different parameters of interest for crops is a useful tool for improving agricultural production (e.g Garcia-Sanchez et al. [4], Zhu et al. [15], Alippi et al. [1]). On these issues, the Wireless Sensor Networks (WSNs) have been proven very useful with high accuracy according to the provided measurements (e.g. Hwang et al. [6], Zhu et al. [15], Garcia-Sanchez et al. [4], Quynh et al. [12]). A wireless sensor network is composed of a number of sensor nodes which usually have small volume, low cost and low power consumption (Zhu et al. [15]). The sensor nodes record data autonomously. The recorded information from the sensors is transmitted to a server and collected in a database for further analysis and/or provision to the users (Fig. 5). Some systems send commands to the nodes in order to fetch the data, while others allow the nodes to send data out autonomously (Hart et al. [5]).

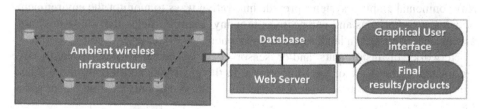

Fig. 5. Generic schematic data flow in an environmental system based on sensor network

5   Variant Scale Ambient Systems

A classical form of ambient systems for the environmental monitoring is the meteorological station networks. Such networks are installed and operate at all scales (from local to global scale) usually through the collaboration among different organizations and institutions (Fig. 6). The recorded data of each of the stations within a network are being transmitted automatically in the central station of the network in order to be validated and/or used for climatological and meteorological analyses. It is mentioned also that these networks are essential to provide with initial conditions the Numerical Weather Prediction (NWP) models that are used for weather forecasting. At this point, it is mentioned that the most commonly used meteorological networks in Greece, belong to the Hellenic National Meteorological Service (www.hnms.gr) and the National Observatory of Athens (www.meteo.gr)

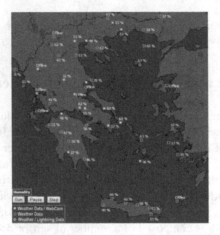

Fig. 6. An example of the several meteorological station networks that operate providing to the public, in real time basis, significant meteorological parameters (http://www.meteogreece.net/)

6   Conclusions

Environmental ambient systems provide innovative ways to monitor the environment, opening new horizons and perspectives in many scientific fields that study the Earth and its characteristics in land, seas and atmosphere.

Networks of instruments and/or sensors can be operated with modern, fully automated methods are of vital importance in the environmental monitoring because can provide on a real time basis accurate information, not only in time but in space too.

As above mentioned, these systems record, collect and monitor specific environmental parameters, more generic parameters like meteorological, or other spatial and temporal parameters. Moreover, after the data storage in a server database, all the collected datasets can be analyzed and/or visualized using a Geographic

Information System (GIS), combined with a satellite image and/or map and published via the Web providing to the users easy access to the relative information.

According to different kinds of monitoring requirements, it can be realized by changing the type of sensors (or instruments) that different environmental issues such as forest fires, agriculture, floods and a vast series of parameters and phenomena can be monitored.

Therefore, such networks of sensors/instruments applied for environment monitoring, play an important role which leads to strengthening the protection of the environment in the near future.

References

1. Alippi, C., Boracchi, G., Camplani, R., Roveri, M.: Wireless sensor networks for monitoring vineyards. In: Anastasi, G., Bellini, E., Di Nitto, E., Ghezzi, C., Tanca, L., Zimeo, E. (eds.) Networked Enterprises. LNCS, vol. 7200, pp. 295–310. Springer, Heidelberg (2012)
2. Bais, A.F., Meleti, C., Kazantzidis, A., Topaloglou, C., Zerefos, C.S., Kosmidis, E.: Greek UV Network: Results and perspectives after three years. In: 8th Conference on Meteorology – Climatology and Atmospheric Physics, Athens, Greece, May 24-25 (2006)
3. Chronis, T., Anagnostou, E.: Evaluation of a Long-Range Lightning Detection Network with Receivers in Europe and Africa. IEEE Transactions on Geoscience and Remote Sensing 44, 1504–1510 (2006)
4. Garcia-Sansez, A.-J., Garcia-Sansez, F., Garcia-Haro, J.: Wireless sensor network deployment for integrating video-surveillance and data-monitoring in precision agriculture over distributed crops. Computer and Electronics in Agriculture 75, 288–303 (2011)
5. Hart, K.J., Martinez, K.: Environmental Sensor Networks: A revolution in the Earth system science? Earth-Science Reviews 78, 178–191 (2006)
6. Hwang, J., Shin, C., Yoe, H.: Study on an Agricultural Environment Monitoring Server System using Wireless Sensor Networks. Sensors 10, 11189–11211 (2010)
7. Kazantzidis, A., Bais, A.F., Topaloglou, C., Garane, K., Zempila, M., Meleti, C., Zerefos, C.S.: Quality assurance of the Greek UV Network: preliminary results from the pilot phase operation. In: Proceedings of SPIE Europe Remote Sensing of Clouds and the Atmosphere XI, Stockholm, Sweden, September 11-14, vol. 6362, pp. 636229-1–636229-10 (2006)
8. Kazantzidis, A., Bais, A.F., Zempila, M., Meleti, C., Eleftheratos, K., Zerefos, C.S.: Evaluation of ozone column measurements over Greece with NILU-UV multi-channel radiometers. International Journal of Remote Sensing 30, 4273–4281 (2009)
9. Kohn, M., Galanti, E., Price, C., Lagouvardos, K., Kotroni, V.: Nowcasting thunderstorms in the Mediterranean region using lightning data. Atmospheric Research 100, 489–502 (2011)
10. Lagouvardos, K., Kotroni, V., Betz, D.-H., Schmidt, K.: A comparison of lightning data provided by ZEUS and LINET networks over Western Europe. Natural Hazards and Earth Systems Sciences 9, 1713–1717 (2009)
11. Mattos, V.E., Machado, L.: Cloud-to-Ground lightning and Mesoscale Convective Systems. Atmospheric Research 99, 377–390 (2011)
12. Quynh, T.N., Vinh, T.T., Quynh, M.B.T.: Multipath routing for cluster-based and event-based protocols in wireless sensor networks. In: 3rd Symposium on Information and Communication Technology, SoICT 2012, Ha Long, August 23-24, pp. 172–179 (2012)

13. Tadesse, A., Anagnostou, E.: Characterization of warm season convective systems over US in terms of CG lightning, cloud kinetics & parameterization. Atmospheric Research 91, 36–46 (2009)
14. Triantafyllou, A.G., Evagelopoulos, V., Zoras, S.: Design of a web-based information system for ambient environmental data. Journal of Environmental Management 80, 230–236 (2006)
15. Zhu, Y., Song, J., Dong, F.: Applications of wireless sensor network in the agriculture environment monitoring. Procedia Engineering 16, 608–614 (2011)

Author Index

Alifragkis, Stavros   1
Angelidis, Pantelis   50, 65
Angelis, Constantinos T.   104
Angelis, Stavros   31

Bagga, Vibhuti   16
Behan, Miroslav   113
Bonnet, Christian   91

Chandra, Sushil   16
Chen, Wei   81

Gavrilis, Dimitris   31

Imadali, Sofiane   65

Kahol, Kanav   16
Kalakos, Nikos   23
Karanasiou, Athanasia   65
Karvounis, Evagelos   41
Koliopanos, Christos   104
Kolios, Stavros   123

Kregting, Wout   81
Krejcar, Ondrej   113

Nakos, Ioannis   41

Papakonstantinou, George   1
Papantoniou, Agis   23
Petrescu, Alexandru   65
Poursanidis, George   50

Sifniadis, Ioannis   65
Smanis, Ioannis   50
Stylios, Chrysostomos   123

Tsalikakis, Dimitrios G.   41, 50
Tsiakalou, Eirini   104
Tsipouras, Markos   41
Tsoulos, Ioannis   31
Tzallas, Alexandros T.   41, 50

Vellidou, Eleftheria   65

Wetterwald, Michelle   91